THE GOOD COOKS COOKBOOK

CLEAN EATING DIET FOR HEALTHY LIVING

It Just Tastes Better!

VOLUME 3 (ANTI-INFLAMMATORY DIET)

COOKING GENIUS
COOKING | KITCHEN

COOKING GENIUS
COOKING | KITCHEN

www.CookingGenius.com

Published by Speedy Publishing LLC

RECIPE CONTENTS

CLEAN EATING AND THE ANTI-INFLAMMATORY DIET: WHY ARE THEY HEALTHY?

You've probably heard of both clean eating and the anti-inflammatory diet before. Maybe you've even been tempted to try them. But do you really understand what these terms mean and why these diets are good for you?

Wonder no more. This article will take you through the basics of both clean eating and the anti-inflammatory diet. Along the way, you'll find out why eating clean could make all the difference in the world to your health.

What Is Clean Eating?

Everyone's heard of clean eating. It's hard to look up any information about nutrition or food without running across this buzzword, and you've probably even heard your family, friends, or coworkers bragging about how they're trying to "eat clean." But what exactly does this mean?

In a nutshell, clean eating means eating minimally-processed foods (or "whole" foods). The closer a food is to its source, the "cleaner" it is. That means fresh vegetables and fruits are great foods to include in a clean diet, because they've remained pretty much unchanged from the time they were picked. Foods like crackers, instant noodles, and baked goods, on the other hand, aren't "clean" at all. They've undergone so much processing that they've become unrecognizable.

A clean diet is, in general, a very healthy diet. That's because minimally-processed foods tend to be rich in the nutrients we need. Besides that, whole foods are often more satisfying and lower in calories than processed foods, so you feel full after eating less. Highly processed foods, by contrast, tend to be high in calories but low in nutrients.

Eating clean isn't difficult to do, but if you've never tried it before, you might not know where to start. That's okay! These simple guidelines will help you get started.

- Choose less processed foods whenever you can. For instance, instead of making white rice for dinner, switch to brown rice, which has undergone less processing.
- Next time you go to the grocery store, shop around the perimeter of the building, where most of the fresh food is. Avoid the central aisles, since the food there tends to be more highly processed.
- Vegetables are one of the cornerstones of a clean diet, so look for ways to incorporate more

of them into your meals. There are plenty of creative ways to add veggies to your food. Try putting shredded veggies into tomato sauce or casseroles, making delicious green smoothies, or experimenting with different salad recipes.

- Avoid processed meats. For instance, natural turkey breast is a much better choice than bologna.
- Aim for balance in your eating habits. Try to incorporate some complex carbs, some protein, and some healthy fat into every meal.
- Stay away from sugar, especially sugary drinks like soda. Drink water and tea instead.

If you stick to a clean diet, you'll feel more energetic, get sick less often, and maybe lose some weight. If you choose the right foods, you could reduce your inflammation, too. Why is that such good news? Keep reading to find out.

What Is Inflammation, and Why Does It Matter?

Inflammation is your immune system's reaction when it thinks your body is being attacked. You can often feel an inflammatory response when you get injured - the affected area might turn red, swell up, and feel warm to the touch. If you've ever gotten a cut or sprained your ankle, you've experienced an inflammatory response. Fever is another type of inflammation.

Inflammation is important, because it's part of how your body defends itself from germs or injuries. But too much inflammation - especially internal inflammation, which you can't feel - can be damaging to your body. Internal inflammation has been linked with numerous diseases, including heart disease, diabetes, and some types of cancer. Inflammation is also associated with a shorter lifespan.

To avoid disease and live a long, healthy life, it's important to keep your inflammation levels as low as possible. That's where the anti-inflammatory diet comes in.

The Anti-Inflammatory Diet and How It Relates to Clean Eating

The amount of inflammation in your body isn't determined by luck or genetics. You can do a lot to control your inflammation levels by simply controlling what you eat. Certain foods lower your inflammation levels, while others can trigger inflammation in your body.

Good news: if you're sticking to a clean diet, you're probably eating lots of anti-inflammatory foods already! There's quite a bit of overlap between clean eating and an inflammation-fighting diet. In general, whole and unprocessed foods tend to lower your inflammation levels, while highly-processed foods increase inflammation (along with your risk of getting sick).

Let's take a look at the foods that are worst for inflammation. For good health, avoid the following:

- Processed sugar
- Trans fats
- White flour
- Alcohol
- Dairy products
- Processed meats

Notice something? With the possible exception of dairy, none of these foods fit into a clean eating plan. When you eat clean, you've already eliminated the worst inflammation-causing foods from your diet.

If you want to lower your inflammation levels while eating clean (and why wouldn't you?), here are some of the best anti-inflammatory foods to incorporate into your diet.

- Dark, leafy greens, such as spinach, kale, and swiss chard
- Wild fish like sardines or salmon
- Flax seeds
- Nuts
- Grass-fed meat (as opposed to grain-fed meat)
- Berries
- Garlic
- Brightly colored veggies, like bell peppers, eggplant, and carrots
- Green tea

The Takeaway

If you want to get healthier, feel better, and live longer, cleaning up your diet is the way to go. Eating clean is simple, delicious, and good for the environment. By eating a clean diet, you'll also reduce your risk of inflammation, which will help you stay healthy as you get older.

Are you inspired to make a change to your diet? How are you going to start eating cleaner today?

SHRIMP SCAMPI

servings: 4 | calories: 276

Ingredients

- 24 large shrimp, peeled and deveined
- 2 tbsps butter
- 2 tbsps olive oil
- 4 small garlic cloves, minced
- 1/8 tsp crushed red pepper flakes
- 1/2 cup dry white wine or broth
- pinch of freshly ground pepper

Directions

1. Melt the butter and olive oil in a large skillet on low heat. Add the garlic and sauté until fragrant. Add the wine or broth, black pepper and red pepper flakes and bring up to a simmer.
2. Add the shrimp and slowly sauté until pink, about two to four minutes for each. Remove from heat and serve immediately.

Shrimp scampi is not only a great dish for dinner, it is also good for you, as shrimp is full of vitamins and protein. Shrimp scampi is also easy to make and is a low fat dish that will please everyone who tries it!

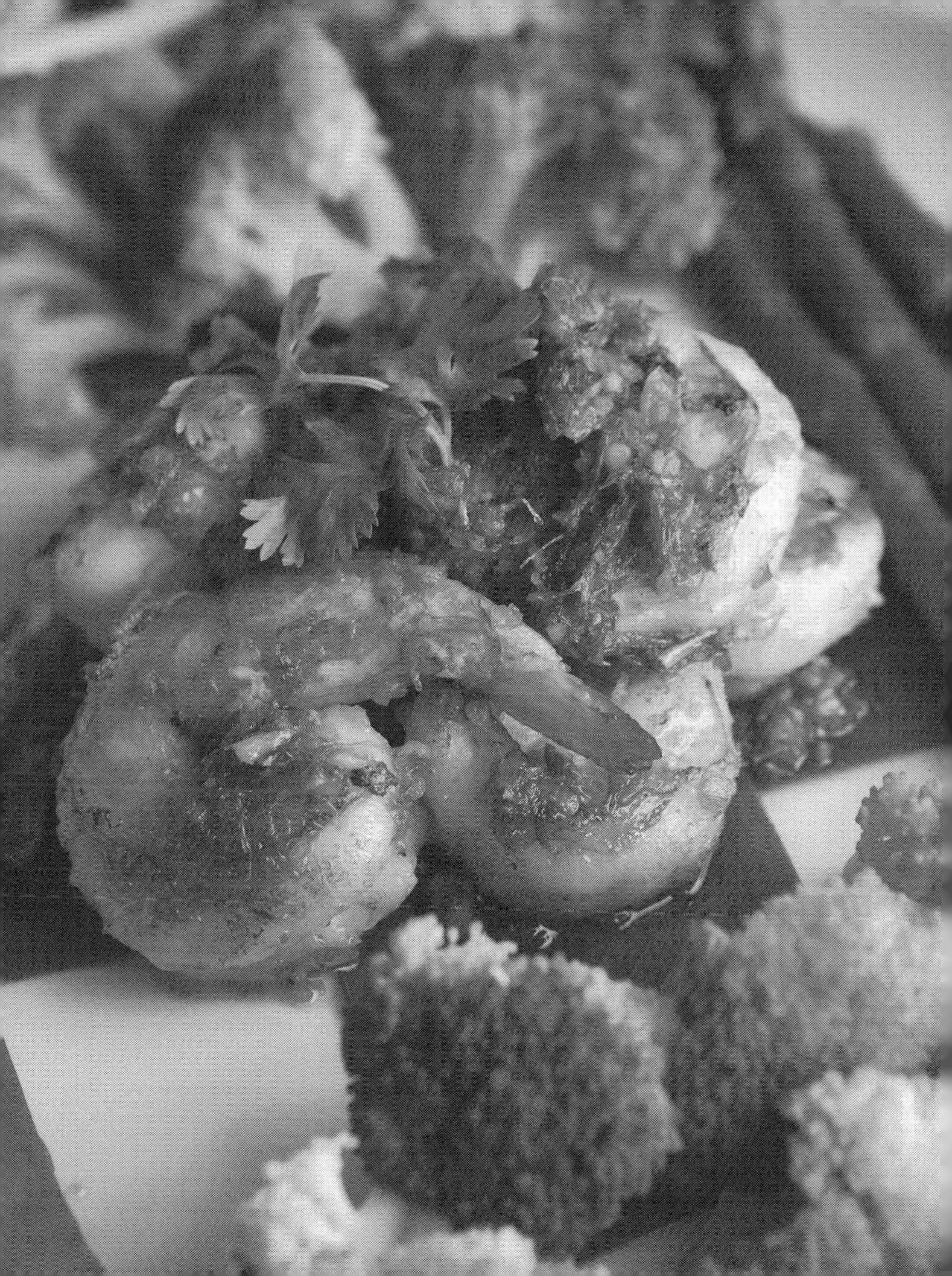

ITALIAN OMELET WITH ZUCCHINI

servings: 2 | calories: 258

Ingredients

- 1/2 cup zucchini, sliced
- 2 onion slices, separated into rings
- 2 tbsp butter
- 3 eggs
- 3 tbsp water
- 1/8 tsp. thyme
- 1/8 tsp. salt
- dash pepper
- 1/4 cup chopped tomato
- 3 tbsp parmesan cheese, shredded

Directions

1. In a 10-inch oven-proof skillet, saute zucchini and onion in butter until crisp tender. Lightly beat eggs, water, thyme, salt and pepper in a small bowl. Pour over zucchini mixture; cook over medium heat. Top set eggs with tomato and cheese; broil until cheese is melted or top lightly browned.

Because high meat consumption can lead to a variety of diseases, meatless dishes are gaining in popularity. Eggs provide high-quality protein and a number of nutrients essential for heart health, while zucchini is an excellent source of fiber, manganese and Vitamin C. Here's a meatless take on a popular breakfast entrée:

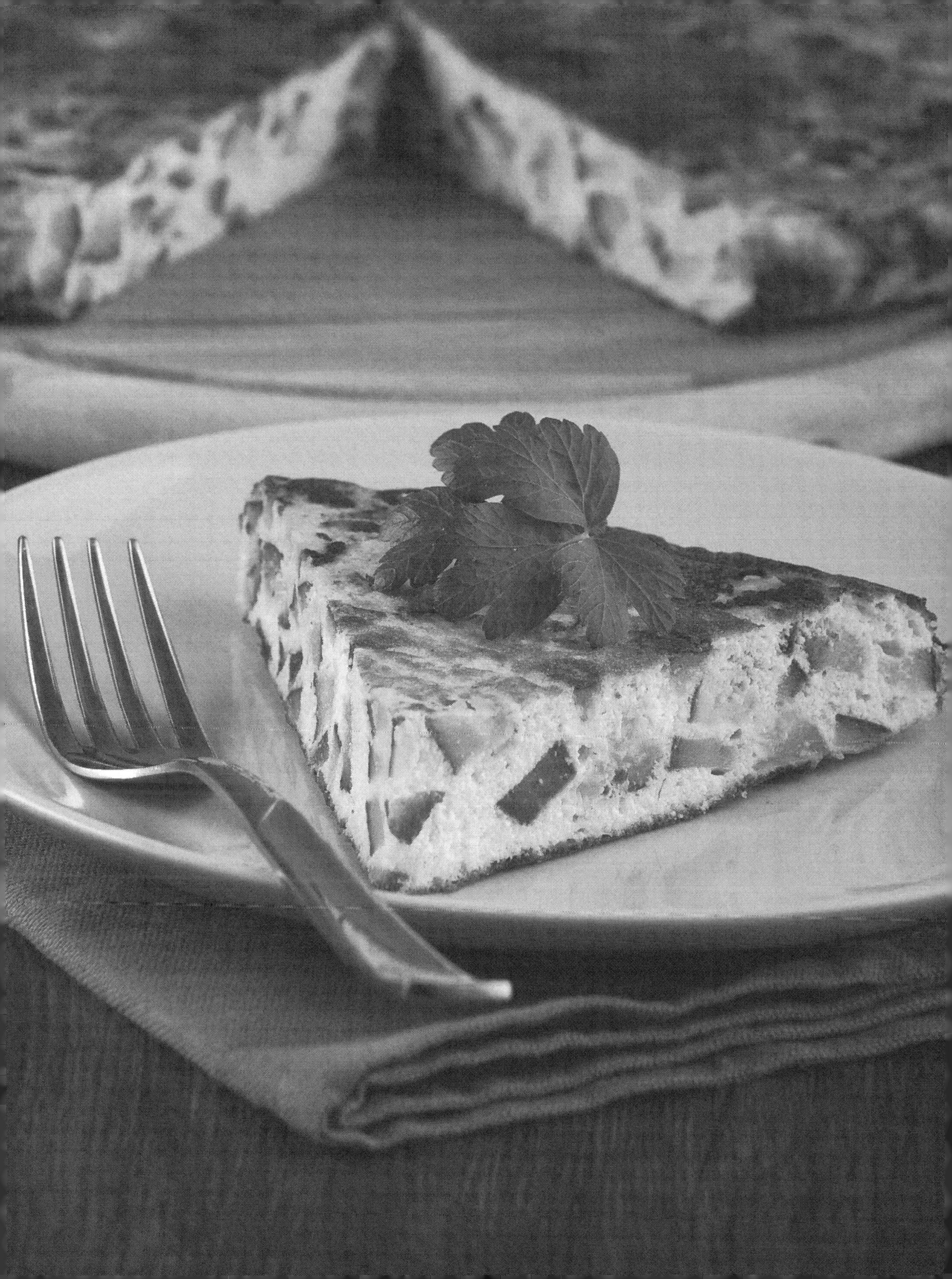

CHILI FRIED CRAB WITH BLACK PEPPER

servings: 3 - 4 | calories: 172

Ingredients

- 3 stone crabs
- oil for frying
- 2 tbsps butter
- 2 garlic cloves, very finely chopped
- 2 tbsps black pepper, ground coarsely
- 10 red or green chilies, chopped
- 2 tbsps soy sauce
- 3 tbsps sugar
- 2 tbsps oyster sauce

Directions

1. Clean the crabs and cut in half. Discard unusable meat from the crab. Smash the claws to allow the seasonings in. Deep fry the crab until half-cooked, drain and set aside.
2. Heat a wok, melt butter and put in garlic, black pepper, and chilies. Saute about 5 to 7 minutes, then add crab and the remaining ingredients. Cook for 5-10 minutes until the crab is done.

This dish has crab, loads of butter, chilies, and black pepper. What's not to like? The preparation and cooking of this dish is also very easy. This recipe will serve 3-4 people depending on the size of the stone crabs.

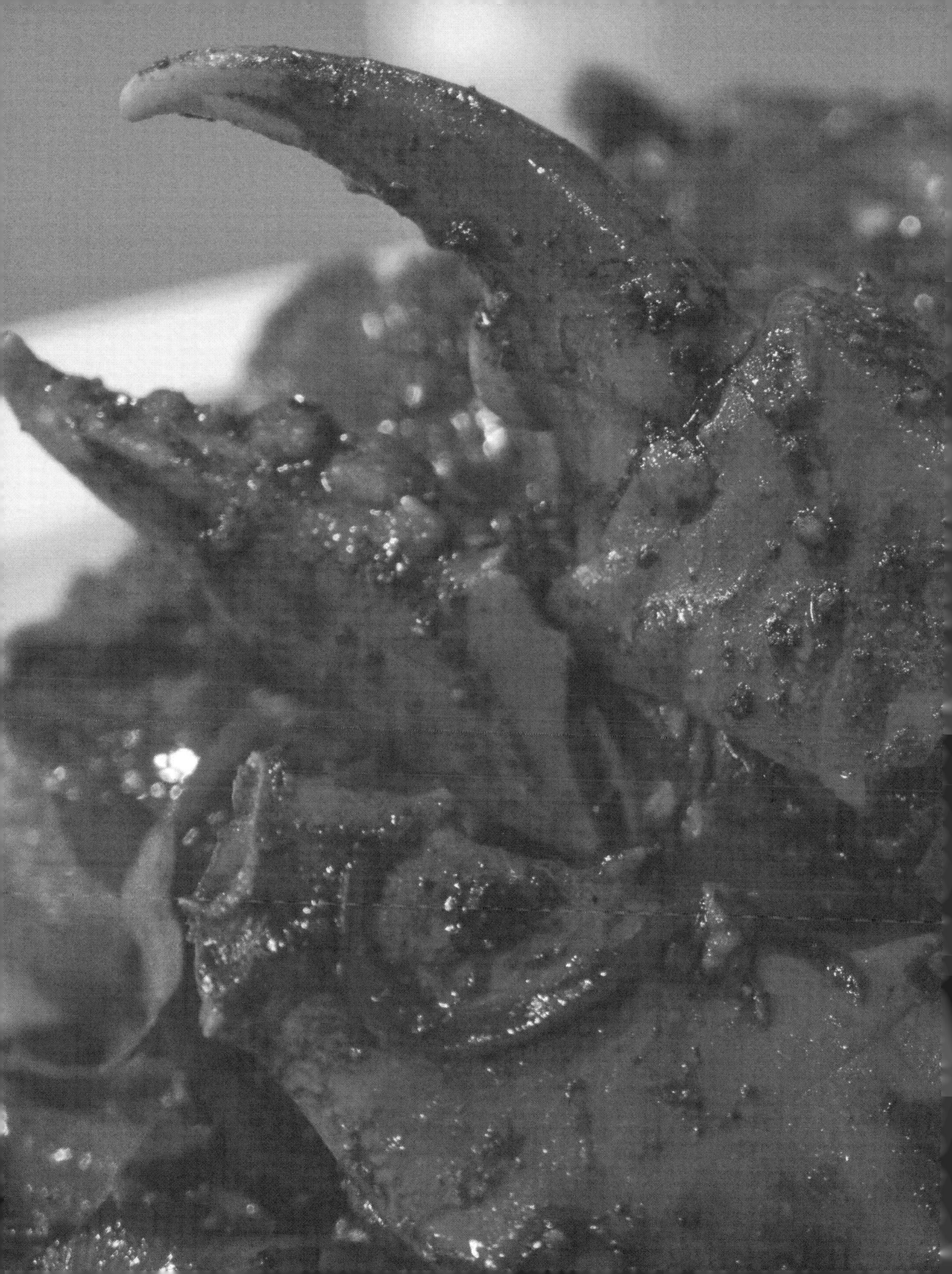

GREEN BEANS, STEWED WITH PANCETTA

servings: 2 | calories: 136

Ingredients

- 2-4 cups of green beans (can vary depending on your family size)
- 2-3 strips of pancetta
- 1 tbsp of butter
- lemon pepper (to taste)

Directions

1. Remove tips from green beans. Break green beans in half. Rinse.
2. Cut pancetta into smaller, quarter length pieces. Set aside.
3. Place green beans in a medium sauce pan.
4. Cover green beans with water until the beans are fully submerged.
5. Place pan over medium-to-high heat on stove. Depending on your stove, heat temperature may vary, adjust accordingly.
6. Add cut up pancetta. Cover.
7. Boil green beans. For al dente, boil for about 8-10 minutes. Softer beans may require more time. Poke with fork to check doneness.
8. Once done, remove pan from heat.
9. Drain beans.
10. Add butter. Add lemon pepper or any other seasoning to taste.
11. Serve immediately and enjoy!

Green Beans are a great side dish to accompany an array of different meals. Green Beans are also a good source of fiber and contain Vitamins A, C, K, and B6. An easy side dish to make that's filled with fiber and vitamins, what more could you ask for?

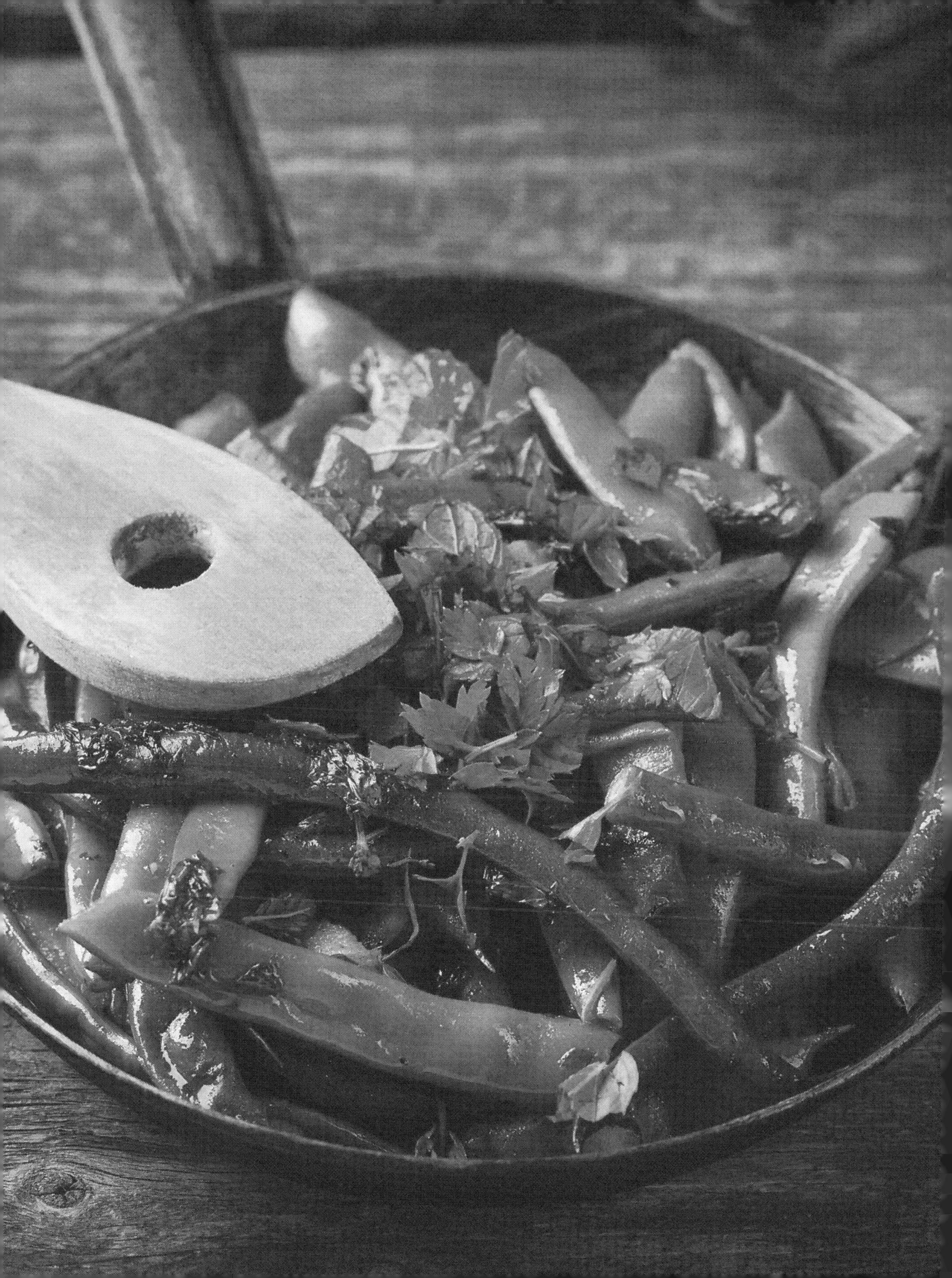

ASPARAGUS WRAPPED IN BACON

servings: 5 | calories: 30 per spear

Ingredients

- 1 bunch asparagus (20 stalks)
- 10 pieces of bacon strips

Directions

1. Wash asparagus and pat dry. Trim off the woody stem - usually the bottom 2 inches.
2. Wrap each spear with a strip of bacon. Place the asparagus on a baking sheet. Place the sheet in the oven that is set to 400 degrees. After about 20 - 25 minutes, check to see that the bacon is cooked.

A delicious way to enjoy this vegetable is to wrap it in bacon. The recipe serves five people and only has a few ingredients, making it a dish that is ideal for an appetizer or a light meal when you don't want to cook.

If you're looking for a vegetable that offers several vitamins and nutrients then consider asparagus. It has a high amount of vitamin K, vitamin E and vitamin C. You can also get large amounts of iron and protein from eating asparagus.

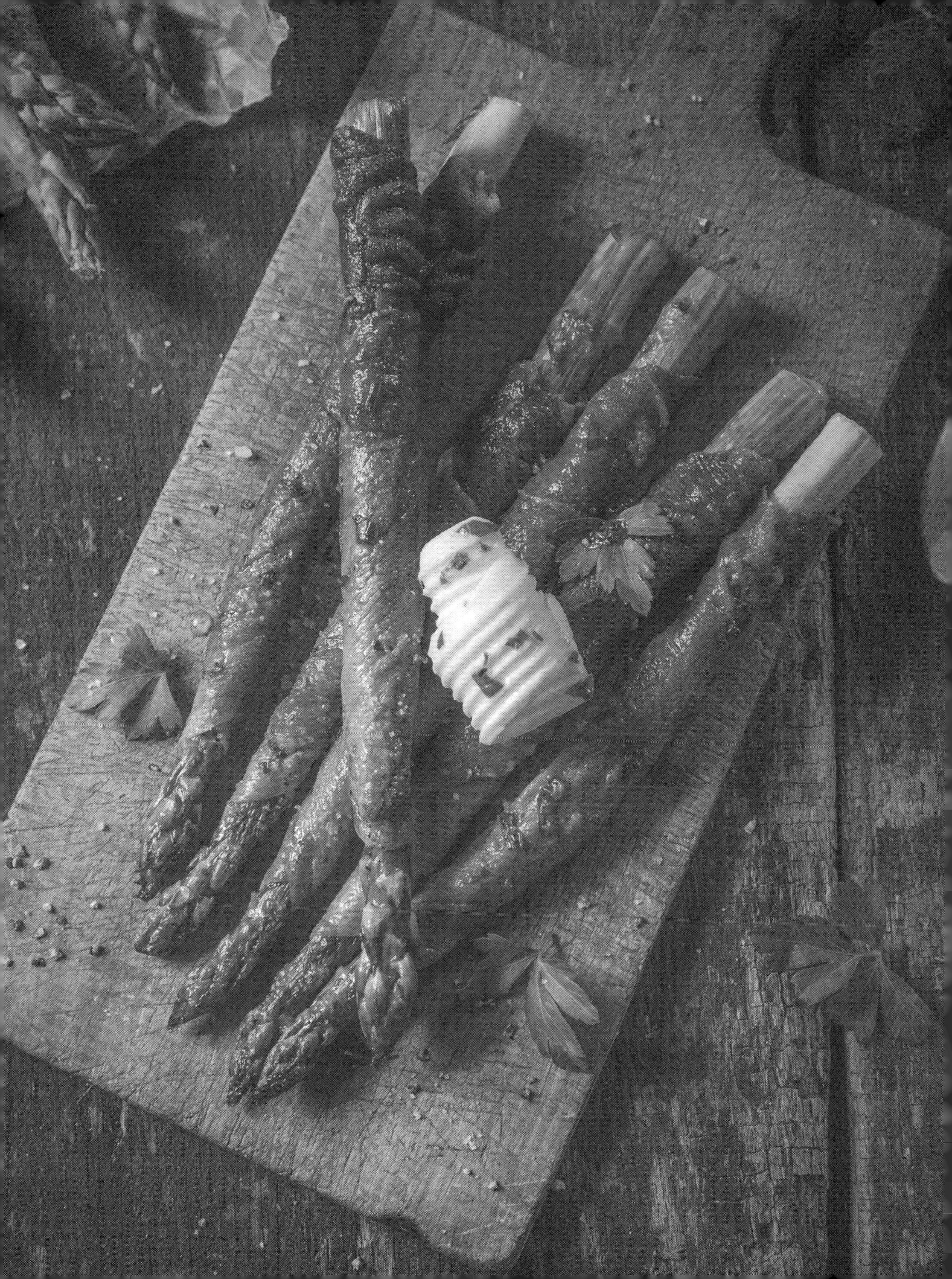

VEAL STEW SOUP

servings: 4 | calories: 464

Ingredients

- 2 lbs of veal
- 1 8-ounce can of tomato sauce
- 1 chopped onion
- 2 cloves garlic, minced
- 1/2 cup of white wine
- 4 tsps olive oil
- salt and pepper to taste

Directions

1. First, take a large pot and heat four teaspoons of olive oil over a medium heat.
2. Add one chopped onion and two cloves of minced garlic to pot, and cook while stirring until the onion is tender.
3. Add two pounds of veal that has been trimmed and cubed to the pot, and let it brown evenly across the meat.
4. Stir in one 8-ounce can of tomato sauce and 1/2 cup of white wine, and season to taste with salt and pepper.
5. Bring the mixture to a boil, and reduce the heat to low, covering the pot and letting it simmer for 90 minutes, or until the meat becomes tender.

Veal is incredibly tasty, but not always easy to make. But with significantly lower amounts of fat and cholesterol to the average cut of beef, veal can give you all the flavor you want with less of the things you don't.

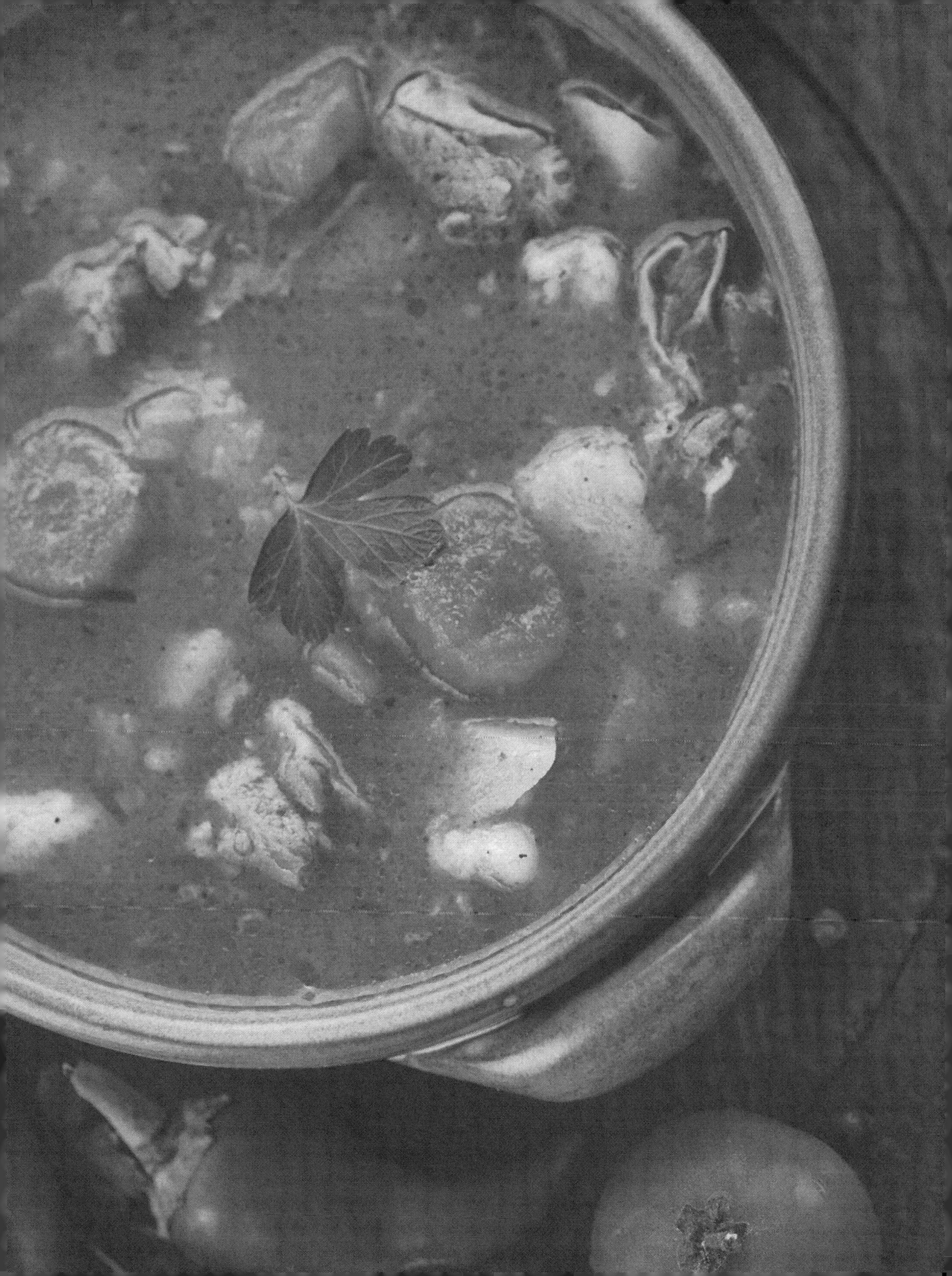

ROASTED LAMB RIBS

servings: 4 | calories: 480

Ingredients

- 1 3/4 lbs lamb ribs
- 1 medium onion, chopped small
- 1/2 cup white wine (dry)
- 1/2 small lemon, squeezed for juice
- 1 tbsp olive oil
- 1 tsp garlic, minced
- 1/2 tbsp honey
- salt and pepper to taste

Directions

1. Decide if you prefer to separate your ribs or keep them in racks (either way works). Place the ribs into a baking dish (approximately 8" x 8" should work; make sure that the pan has at least a ½" in height).
2. In a medium mixing bowl, combine your liquids (wine, lemon juice, olive oil, and honey). Add in your garlic and salt and pepper (use sparingly at first, you can add salt and pepper if needed later). Mix until well blended.
3. Pour mixture over the ribs. Place in refrigerator for 45 minutes to marinate. Preheat the oven to 400. Allow for an additional 5-10 minutes of marinating while oven is heating. Once heated, place on middle rack and allow to cook until browned.
4. Cook time is approximately 60-75 minutes depending on rib size and if you separated ribs.
5. Serve over jasmine or white rice with a touch of drippings for gravy. Enjoy!

Delicious and tender, this incredible roasted lamb recipe is quick and easy to make. Lamb is very high in omega 3 fatty acids as well as protein, both of which are essential to a healthy diet. With a few veggies and a little time, you can quickly prepare this delectable dish.

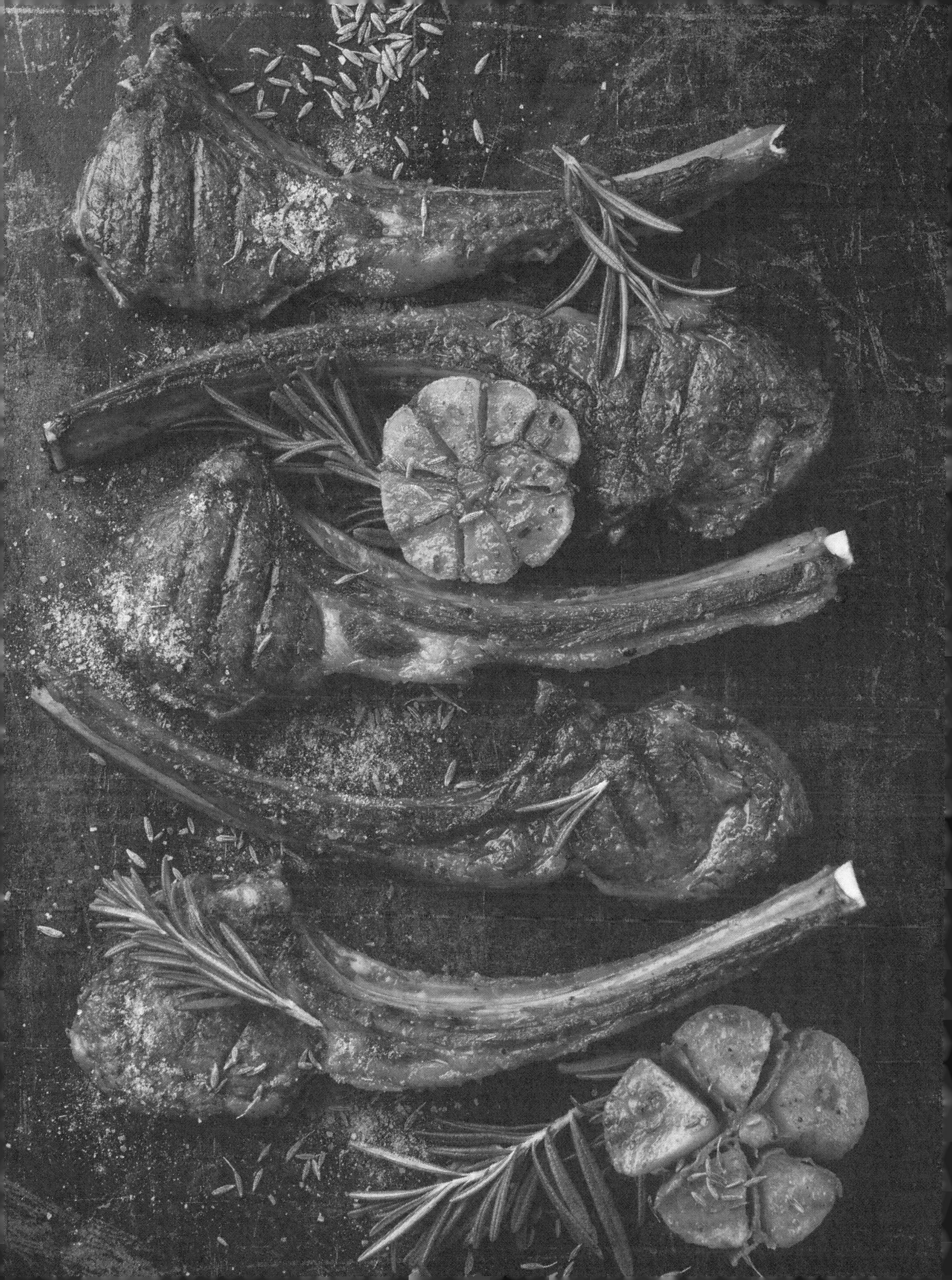

GRILLED RIB EYE STEAK

servings: 4 - 6

Ingredients

- 2 20 ounce rib eye steaks
- kosher salt
- freshly-ground black pepper
- granulated garlic

Directions

1. Remove the steaks from the refrigerator an hour before grilling. Season them on all sides with kosher salt, black pepper and granulated garlic. Sprinkle on olive oil and rub into the meat.
2. Allow the steaks to rest and absorb the seasonings. Turn them every 15 minutes.
3. The grill needs to reach 500F before you start grilling. 30 minutes beforehand might be the best time to light the charcoal.
4. When the grill reaches 500F put the steaks on the grill. Close the lid and set a timer for 2 minutes. After that time, turn the steaks at a 45-degree angle to make sear marks. Close the lid and set the timer for another 2 minutes.
5. After two minutes, flip the steaks to the other side and repeat the process. After 8 minutes, you will have beautifully grilled medium-rare rib eye steaks. Allow the meat to rest for 5-7 minutes before serving.
6. Add an additional 2 minutes for medium. 4 minutes for medium-well done.

The protein in this steak will help fuel your body's metabolism.

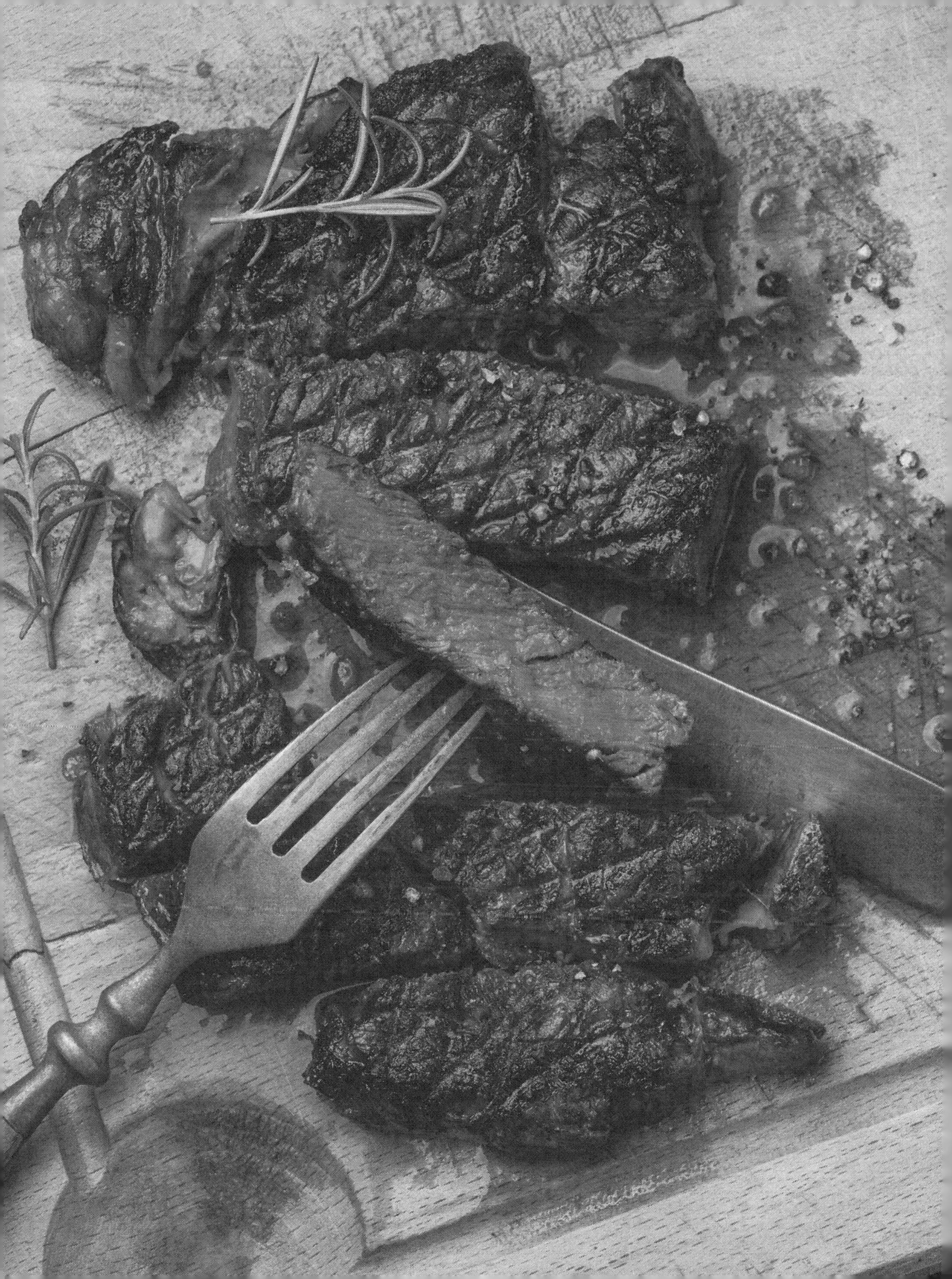

GRILLED VEAL LOIN STEAK MEAT WITH ASPARAGUS AND CHERRY TOMATOES

servings: 4 | calories: 250

Ingredients

- 4 12-ounce veal loin
- 2 tbsps extra-virgin olive oil, plus more for drizzling
- 2 garlic cloves, minced
- 1 tbsp rosemary leaves
- 1/4 cup sage leaves
- 1 bunch asparagus
- 1 1/2 lbs cherry tomatoes
- salt and pepper

Directions

1. Wash and pat dry tomamtoes and asparagus. Trim off the wooded ends of the asparagus.
2. In a small bowl mix 2 tbsps of olive oil with the garlic, rosemary and sage and set aside . Seson the veal with salt and pepper then pour olive oil/herb mixture over it before slowly grilling over a moderately high heat turning to the other side, browning both sides about 6 minutes before lowering the heat and adding the asparagus and tomatoes.
3. Remove the asparagus when they are tender and golden brown from the oil. Slice the tomatoes or leave them whole for a fresh meal idea.

Asparagus is a green vegetable that is full of iron and vitamin K. Potassium and zinc are also found in asparagus. Cherry tomatoes have high amounts of fiber to keep the digestive system regulated and vitamin C. Veal is a meat that has a high amount of protein and little fat. Grilled veal loin with asparagus and cherry tomatoes is a delicious dish. Grilling the meat and the vegetables will help to lock in the flavors and the nutrients.

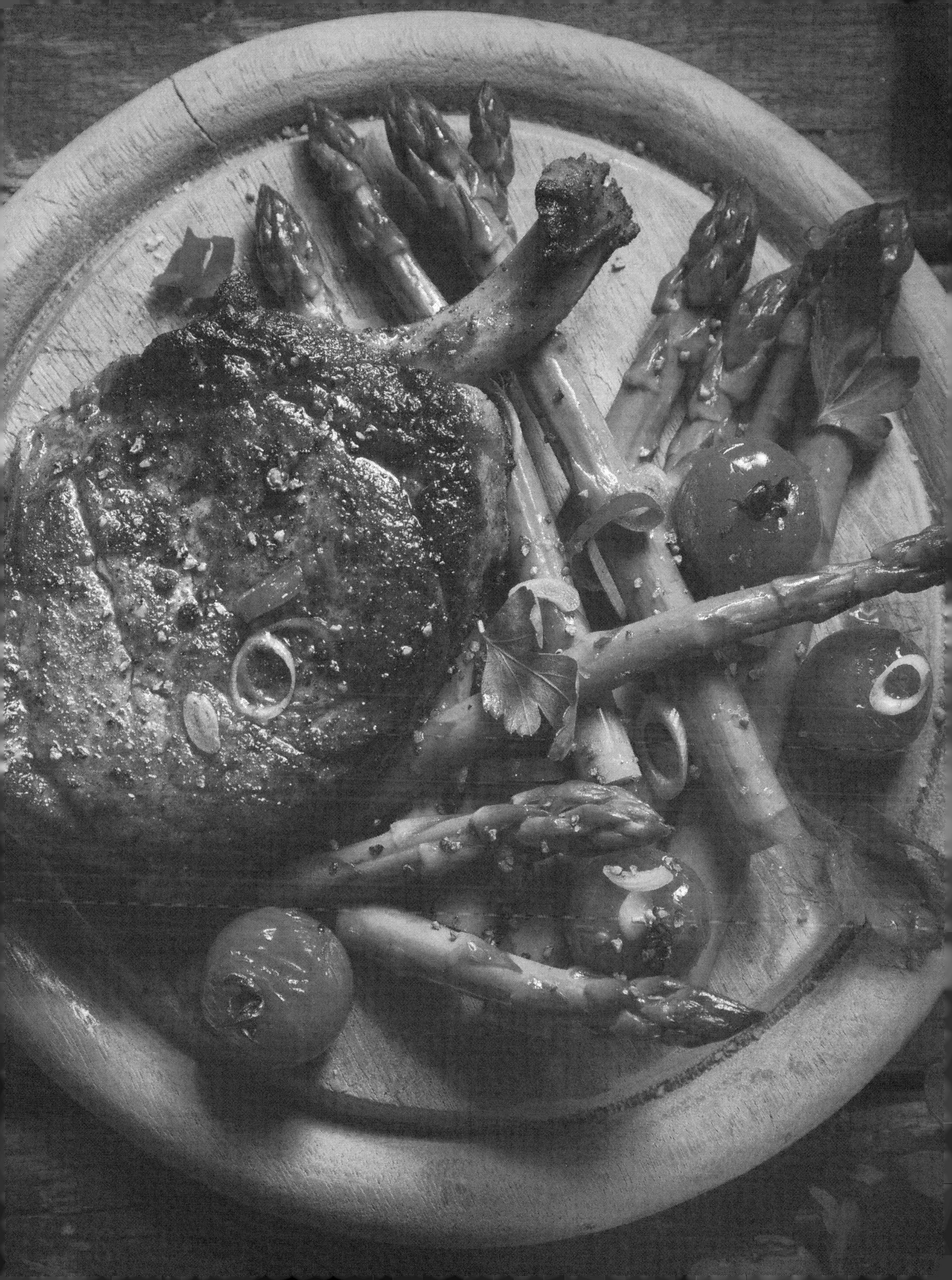

GRILLED TERIYAKI SALMON STEAK GARNISHED WITH GRILLED PINEAPPLE, BABY EGGPLANTS, ZUCCHINI AND CHILI PEPPER

servings: 4 | calories: 480

Ingredients

- 3lbs fresh salmon, bones removed
- 1 pineapple spear
- 1 - 2 baby eggplants
- 1 zucchini
- 1 chili pepper
- 1/3 cup of soy sauce
- 1/3 cup water
- 1 tbsp apple cider vinegar
- 3 tbsp olive oil
- 1 tbsp brown sugar
- 1 garlic clove, minced
- salt and pepper

Directions

1. Cut salmon into four equal pieces. Season with salt and pepper to taste and set aside.
2. In a bowl, combine soy sauce, water, apple cider vinegar, olive oil, brown sugar, and garlic. Stir until the sugar has dissolved, then place salmon and marinade into a plastic bag. Place in refrigerator and allow to marinate for at least half an hour.
3. Meanwhile, slice the vegetables into one-inch cubes and place on skewer. Season with salt, pepper, and oil.
4. After the fish is done marinating, preheat grill to medium heat and lightly oil the grates.
5. Place the salmon on one side of the hot grill, discarding marinade. On the other side of the grill, place down vegetable skewers.
6. Cook salmon for four to six minutes per side, depending on thickness, or until the fish flakes easily with a fork. Cook vegetables for the same amount of time.
7. Remove salmon and vegetables from grill. Allow fish to rest for five minutes before serving.

Nothing quite says summer like grilled teriyaki salmon, that perfect complement of salty and sweet. Add a garnish of grilled pineapple, baby eggplants, zucchini and chili pepper, and you have a healthful meal filled with heart-healthy omega-3 fatty acids, protein, and B vitamins.

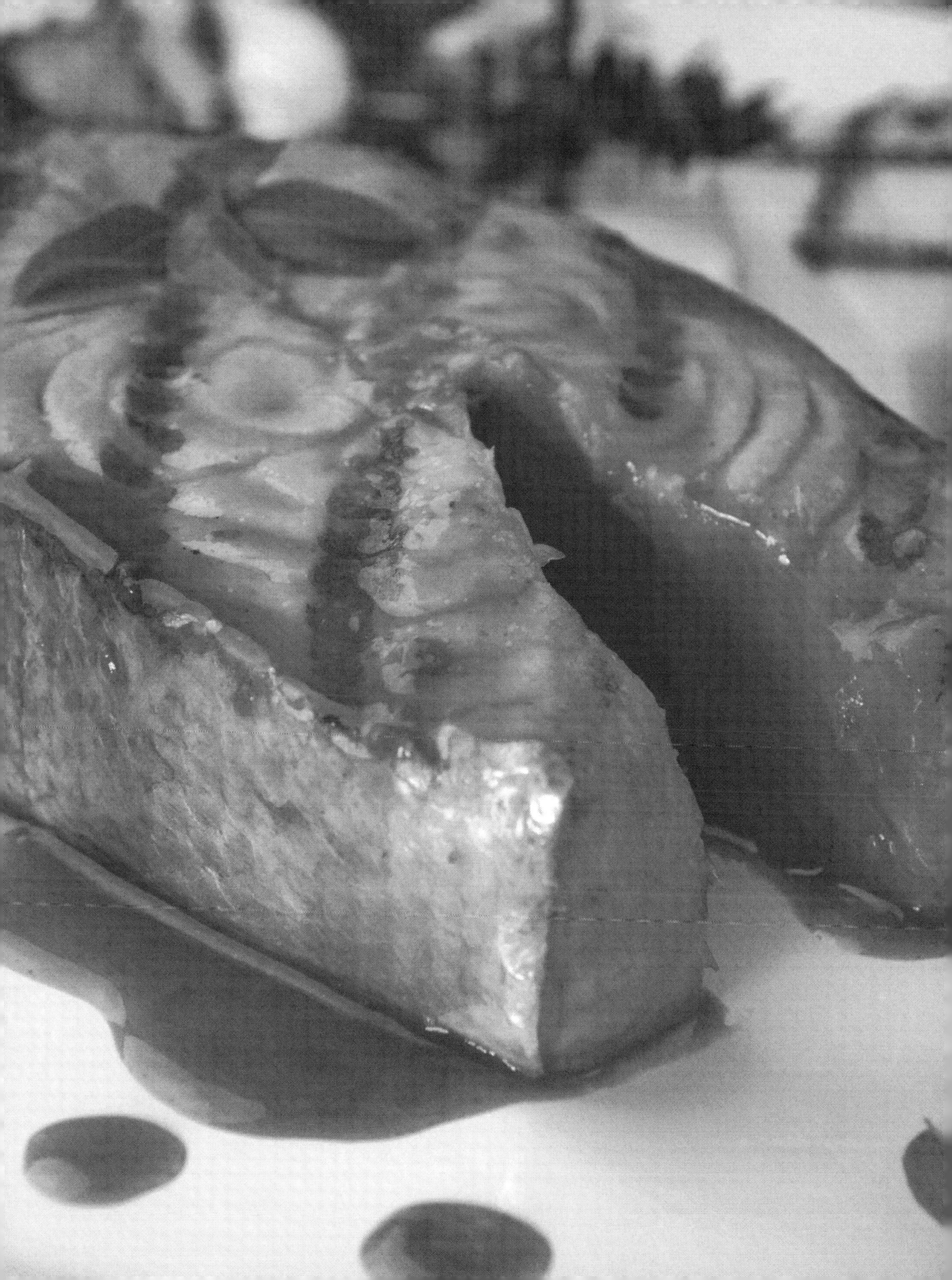

MUSHROOM QUICHE

servings: 6 - 8 | calories: 301

Ingredients

- 4 cups sliced mixed mushrooms, shiitake, oyster and portobello
- 1 1/2 cups grated cheddar
- 1 tbsp olive oil
- 1 small red onion, thinly sliced
- 1/2 tsp dried thyme
- 1/4 tsp dried basil
- 1/4 tsp dried rosemary
- 3 eggs
- 1 cup heavy cream or milk
- 1/4 tsp salt
- pinch of pepper
- pinch of nutmeg
- frozen puff pastry, thawed

Directions

1. Preheat oven to 400°F
2. Roll out the pastry on a lightly floured surface until it's slightly larger than your baking dish. Press the pastry into the pan. Trim the edges. Evenly cover the pastry with the grated cheese and place in the refrigerator.
3. Over medium-high heat, saute the onions and mushrooms in the olive oil, stirring regularly until they have cooked down and the liquid has disappeared. Stir in thyme, rosemary and basil. Remove from the heat and allow to cool slightly.
4. Whisk the eggs and milk together. Add the salt, pepper and nutmeg. Bring out the baking dish. Spread the mushroom mixture over the cheese. Add the egg mixture.
5. Bake 35-40 minutes until a knife inserted in center comes out clean. Serve warm.

Mushroom Quiche is perfect for any meal or as a side dish.

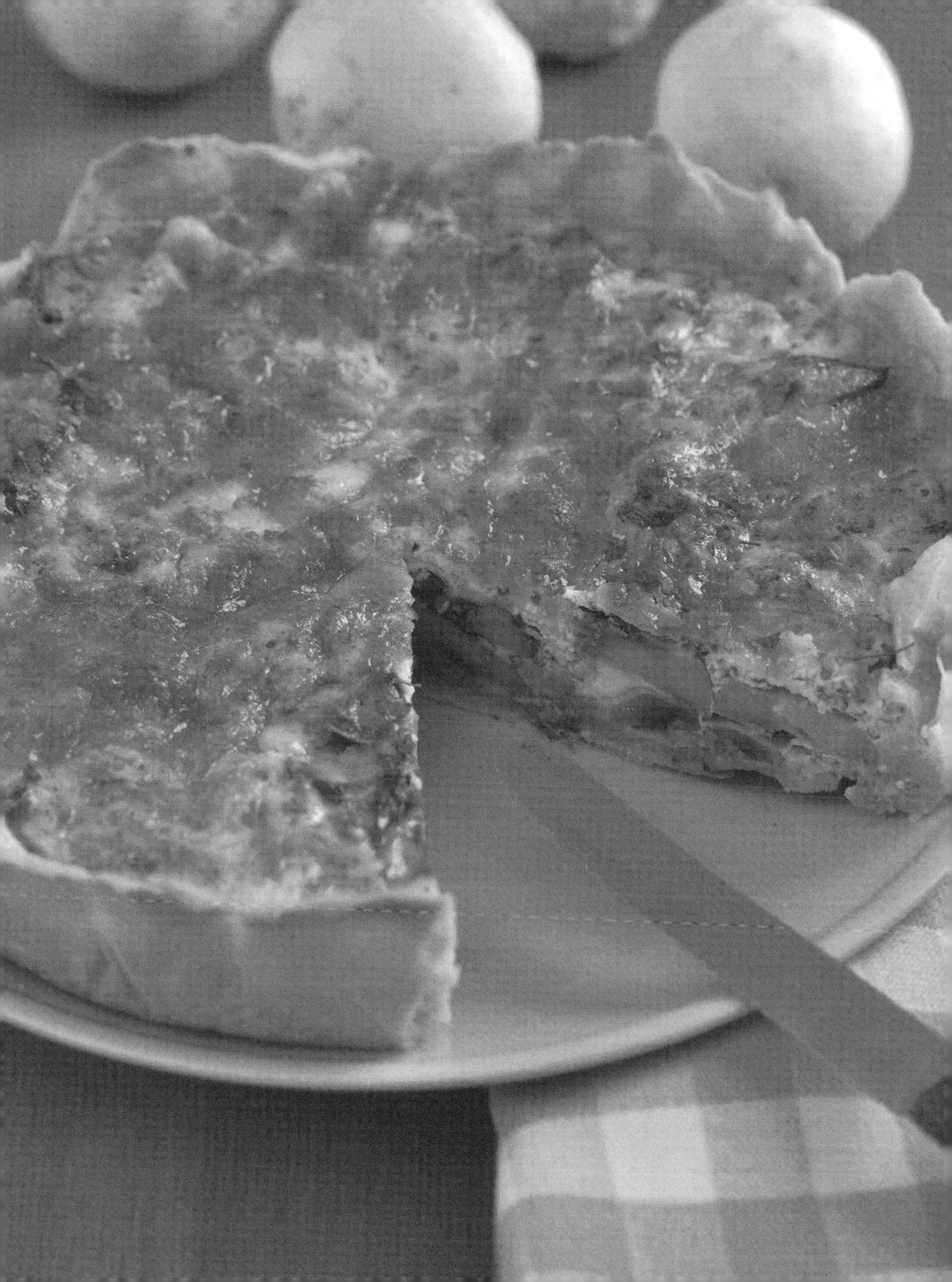

STUFFED PEPPERS WITH MINCED MEAT (BEEF), CHEESE AND FRESH HERBS

servings: 6 | calories: 418

Ingredients

- 6 green bell peppers (large)
- 1 lb. ground beef
- ½ cup onion (chopped)
- 1 16 oz. can diced tomatoes (drained)
- 1 cup long grain rice (cooked)
- 1 cup water
- 1 tsp salt
- 1 tsp worcestershire sauce
- 1 cup cheddar cheese (shredded)
- 2 tbsps parsley (minced)

Directions

1. Heat oven to 350 degrees.
2. Bring a large pot of water to boil.
3. Prep the peppers. Cut off the tops of the green peppers about ¼ inch from stem. Reserve. Remove and discard seeds and membranes. Place the peppers into the boiling water to soften the skin, about 5 minutes.
4. Use the reserved tops and mince peppers leaving the stem behind. Remove peppers from boiling water and place on a wire rack to drain.
5. Prepare the filling. In a skillet cook ground beef, onion, minced peppers, and ½ tsp. salt. Drain off fat, then add tomatoes, salt, Worcestershire, and pepper to taste. Combine meat, rice, ½ the cheese, and herbs
6. Sprinkle the interior of the peppers with salt before stuffing. Divide the filling among the peppers.
7. Place into a baking dish and top with remaining cheese.
8. Cover baking dish with foil and bake 20 minutes. Remove foil and bake for 10 additional minutes.
9. Let stand for 5 minutes before serving.

Stuffed Bell Peppers are great for a crowd or an easy weeknight meal. Delicious and healthy for you--bell peppers are low in calories and high in Vitamins A & C.

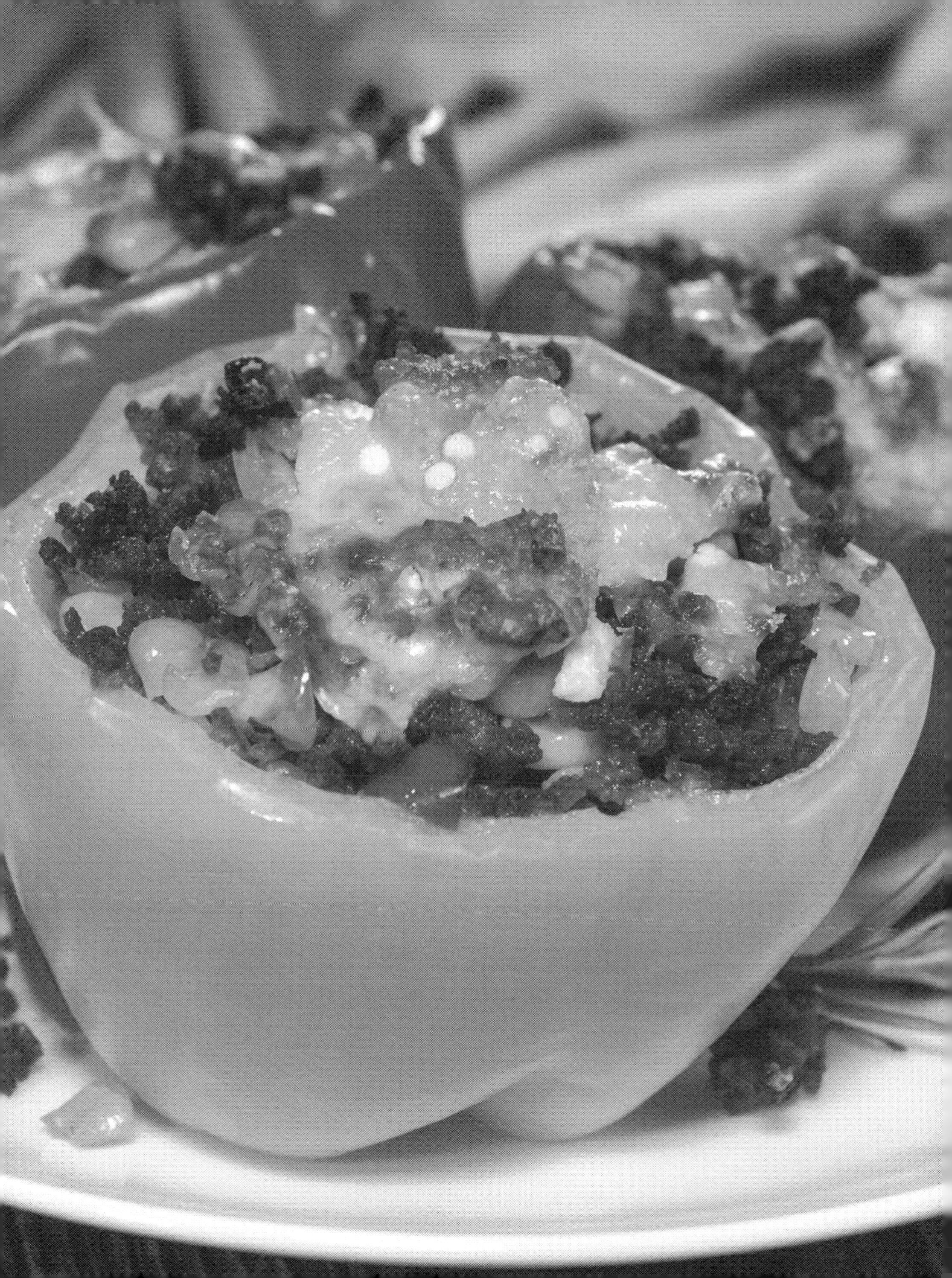

HOMEMADE SPICY DEVILED EGGS WITH PAPRIKA

servings: 2 | calories: 130

Ingredients

- 1/4 cup of mayo
- 1 tsp dijon mustard
- 1 tbsp sriracha (or favorite hot sauce)
- 1/4 tsp black pepper
- 1/4 tsp salt
- 1 tbsp chopped chives
- 1/8 teaspoon paprika
- 1 or 2 slices of cooked bacon strip, crumbled
- 6 large eggs

Directions

1. Place you eggs in a pot that is filled with cold water approx. one inch over eggs. Bring water to boil and cover for 15 minutes. Strain and set eggs aside.
2. Once cooled, peel eggs and slice, scooping out innards and placing them in a bowl. Mash yolk and add mayo, mustard, pepper and salt. Combine well.
3. Squirt 1/4 tsp of hot sauce into each empty egg half. Place sizable scoops of mixture into centers of egg whites. Top with chives, bacon, and paprika.

This recipe yields 6 servings and each serving is 2 deviled eggs. Eggs are a wonderful source of lean protein, which is great for those who are on a diet.

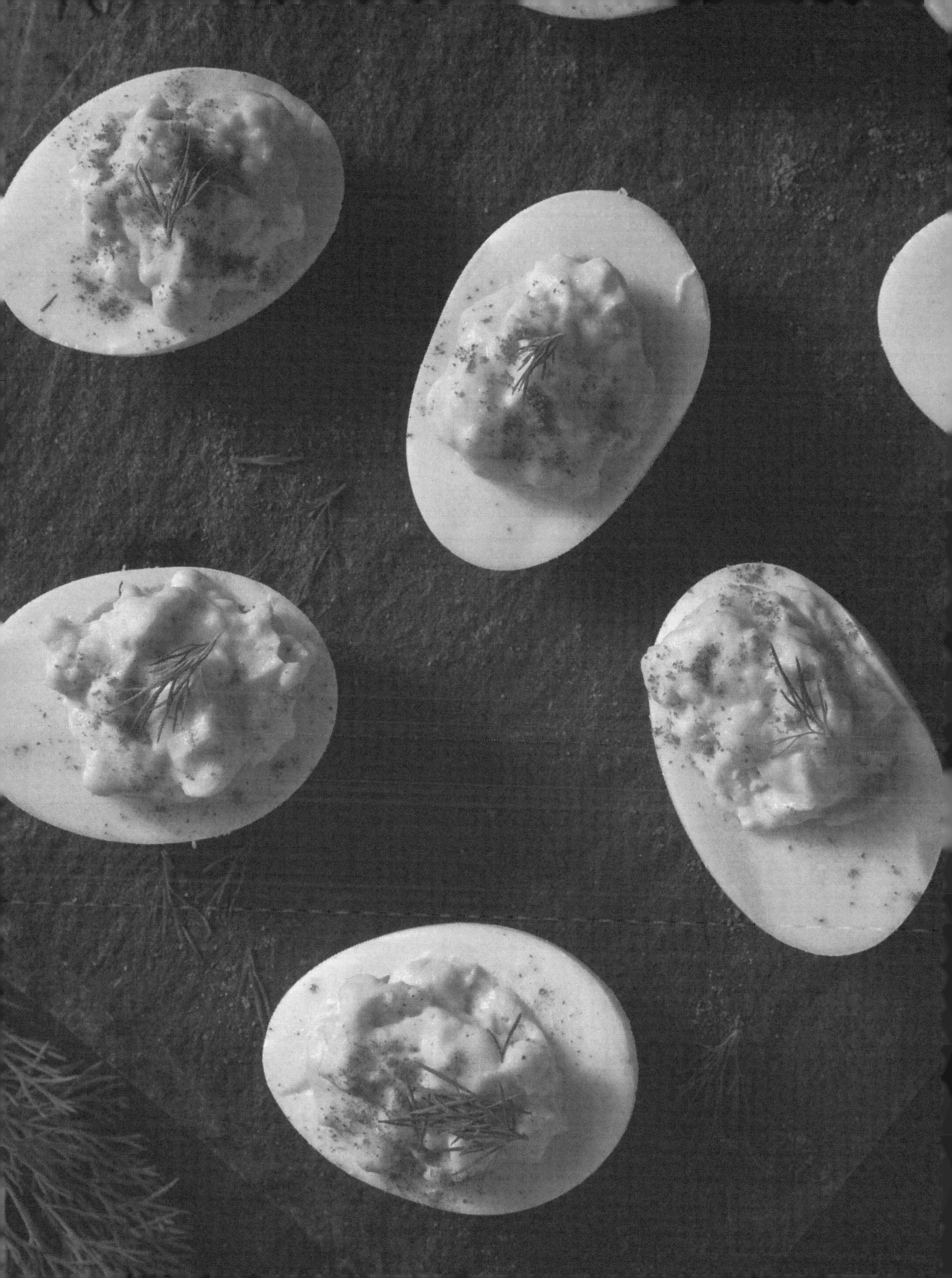

MINI FRITTATAS WITH SMOKED HAM, PEAS, GREEN ONION AND FETA

servings: 12 | calories: 100

Ingredients

- 6 whole eggs
- 2 tablespoons milk
- 3 tablespoons green onions
- 1/4 cups cooked peas
- 3/4 cups cubed smoked ham
- 3/4 cups cheddar cheese
- 1/4 cup feta crumbled cheese
- salt and pepper to taste

Directions

1. Preheat oven to 375 degrees.
2. Grease muffin tins with cooking spray.
3. In one bowl, beat eggs and milk until well blended. Stir in onions and peas/salt and pepper to taste.
4. In a second bowl, mix cubed ham, cheddar, and feta cheese.
5. Divide ham and cheese among 12 muffin tins evenly. Layer egg mixture on top of meat and cheese. Bake 15 – 20 minutes or until center is solid. You can test the center by using a tooth pick or butter knife – insert in the center and if comes out clean, it is fully baked.

This mini frittata is great choice for a quick breakfast or weekend brunch. At approximately 100 calories per serving and loaded with protein, this make ahead breakfast mini is great on the go, but also good for you.

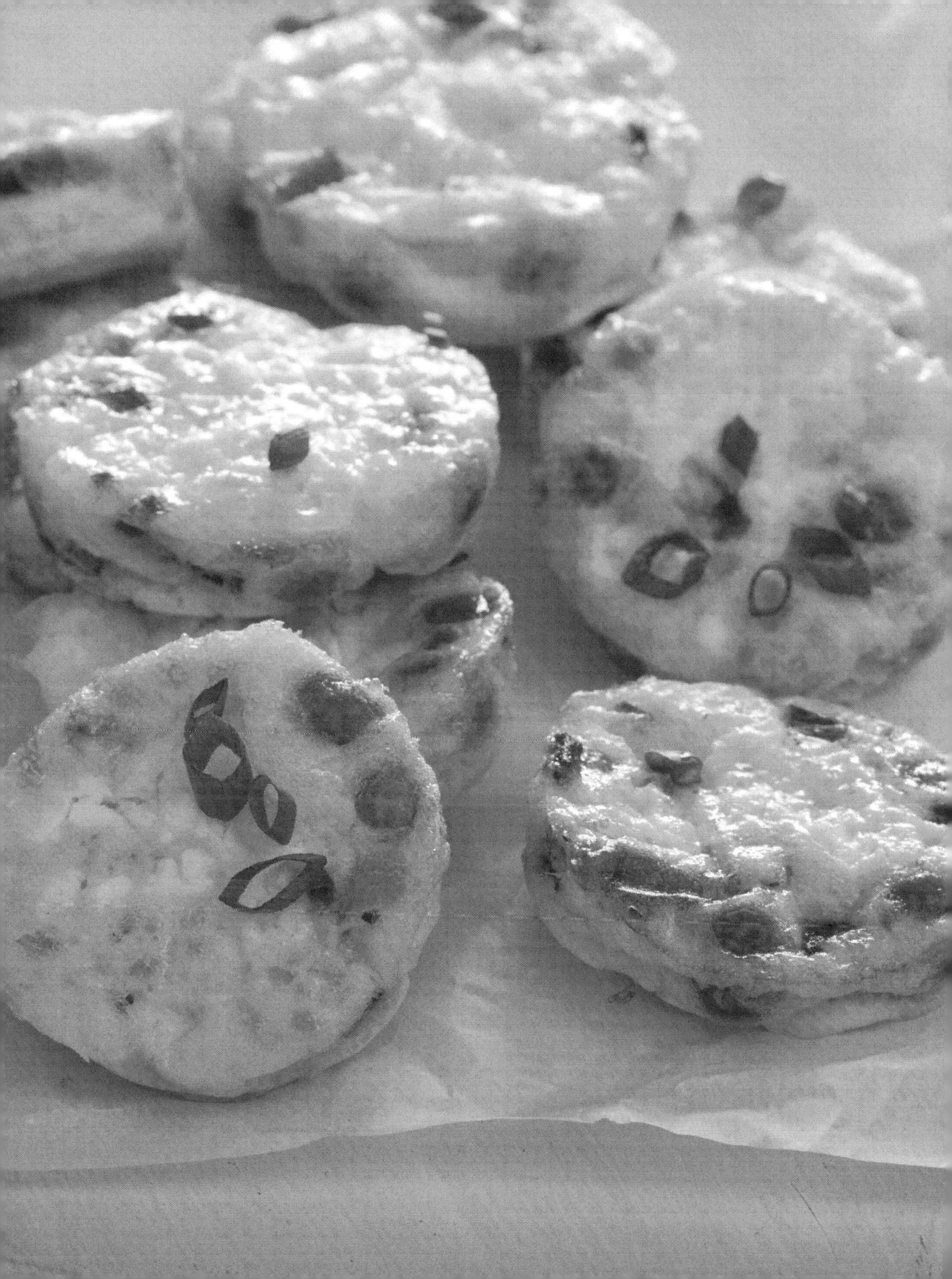

GRILLED VEGETABLES SALAD WITH ZUCCHINI, EGGPLANT, ONIONS, PEPPERS AND TOMATO

servings: 6

Ingredients

- 1 small eggplant, trimmed and cut into bite-size pieces
- 16 cherry tomatoes, cut in half
- 1 medium red onion, cut into rings, cut in half
- 1 yellow and 1 red bell pepper, quartered, removing seeds and ribs
- 1 medium zucchini sliced
- 1/4 cup extra virgin olive oil
- 1/4 cup fresh basil leaves
- 1/4 lb crumbled feta cheese
- salt and freshly ground black pepper

Directions

1. Place all veggies in a bowl and sprinkle with salt, pepper and oil and stir to coat. Place veggies on grill for 5-7 minutes or grill in oven at 425 degrees for 8-12 minutes
2. Dressing: While grilling, mix in small bowl: 1 medium clove chopped garlic, 1 tablespoon balsamic vinegar, 3 tablespoons oil and salt and freshly ground black pepper. Set aside.
3. Place veggies on a platter. Sprinkle with basil leaves and feta. Drizzle dressing over the top. The rainbow colored vegetables add many nutrients, and a bowl of Quinoa on the side will add protein.

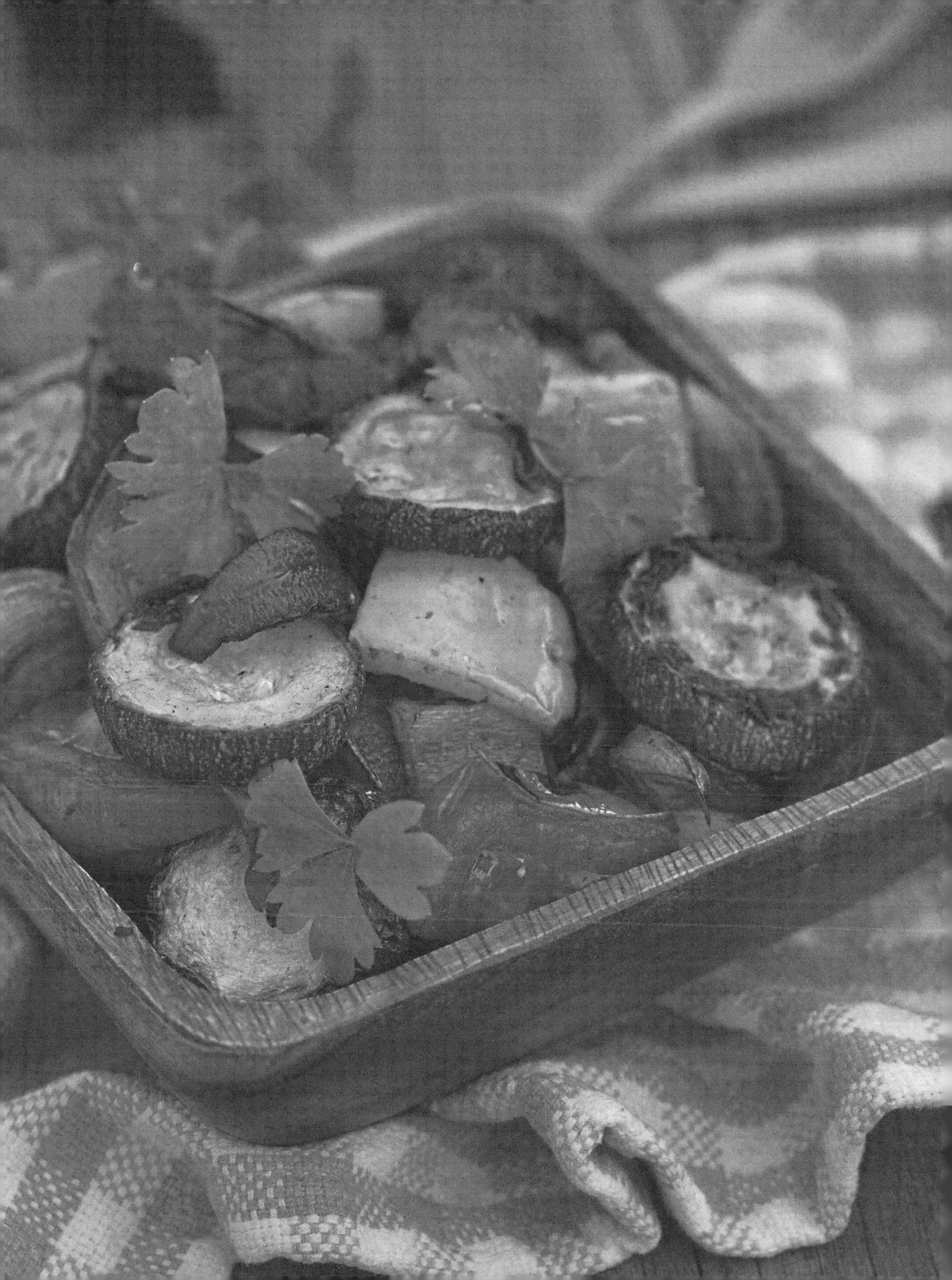

AVACADO AND TOMATO SALAD WITH ONIONS

servings: 6 - 8

Ingredients

- 2 avocados, peeled and cut into bite-sized chunks
- 3-4 large tomatoes, sliced
- 2 tbsps extra virgin olive oil (the best quality)
- 2 tbsps red wine vinegar (a good, strong red wine vinegar)
- 1 teaspoon crumbled dried oregano, or 1 tbsp chopped fresh oregano
- 1 garlic clove, minced
- 1/4 cup chopped fresh parsley
- 1/2 red onion, thinly sliced
- kosher salt
- freshly ground black pepper

Directions

1. The first step to making this delicious meal is to combine the tomatoes, avocados, garlic, parsley, onions, and oregano onto a service platter. Put a layer of tomatoes on the bottom, and then spread the avocados and onions on top of it. Sprinkle the other three on top of them.
2. Use the olive oil and red wine vinegar as a dressing, and then sprinkle a little some salt and freshly ground pepper on top.

This is a quick and easy dish that is a unique and different take on delicious vegetables. This recipe serves 6-8 people, and it can be served immediately or after a while at being at room temperature. However, you never want to put it in the refrigerator.

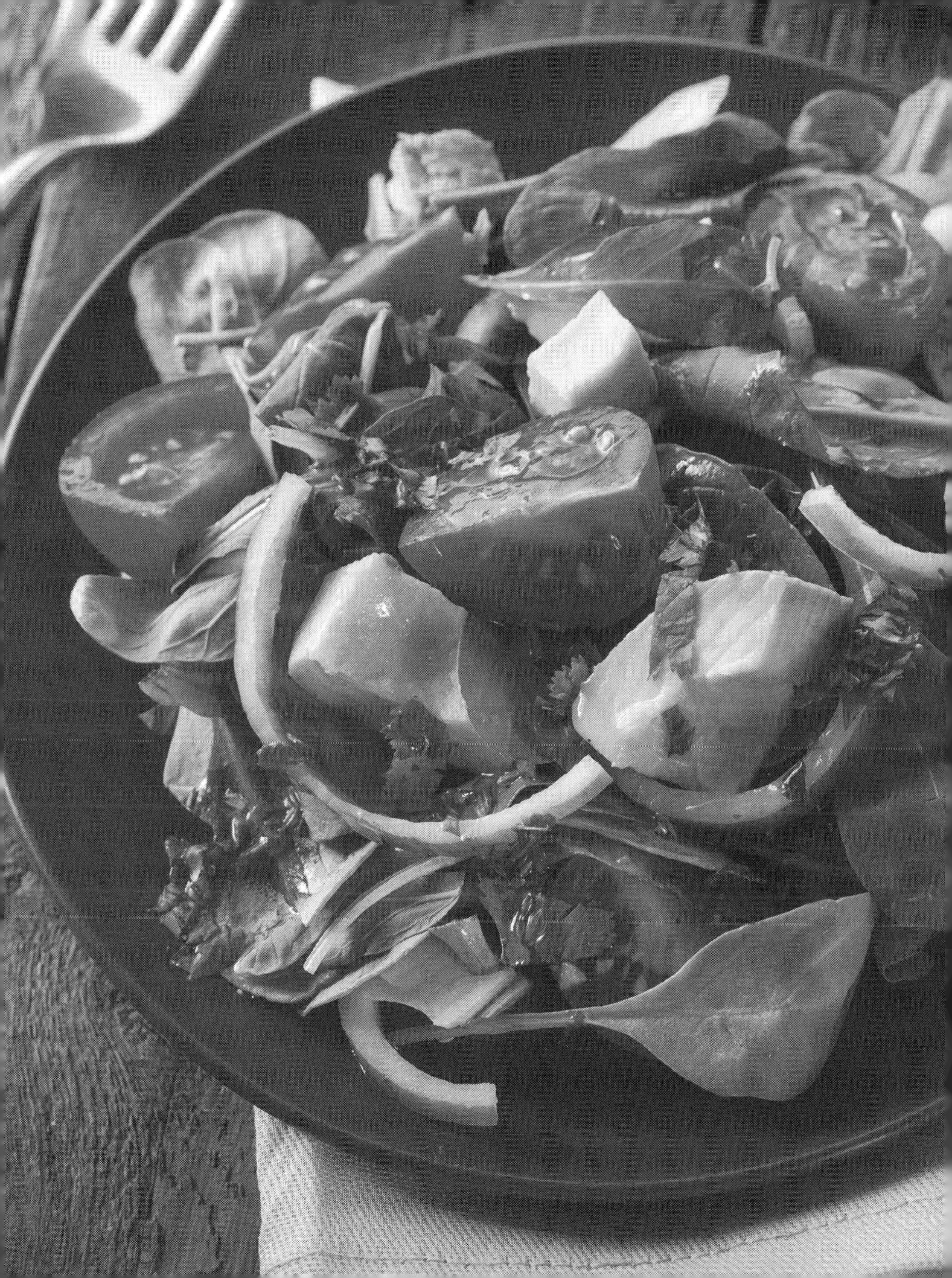

CUCUMBER SALAD

servings: 4 | calories: 33

Ingredients

- 2 english cucumbers, peeled, halved and sliced
- 1/2 a red onion, thinly sliced
- 2 tablespoons chopped dill
- 1/4 cup white wine vinegar
- 2 teaspoons sugar (or stevia)
- sea salt
- pepper

Directions

1. Whisk together the white wine vinegar, sugar and a generous pinch of sea salt and pepper in a large bowl. Add sliced English cucumbers, red onion, and chopped dill. Mix well and cover. Chill in the refrigerator for half an hour before serving.
2. Want an easy twist on this salad? Add two tablespoons of dijon mustard, half a teaspoon of red pepper flakes, or a couple of spoonfuls of crumbled feta cheese.

In the midst of summer we all crave something light and refreshing. Packed with vitamin K, vitamin C and fiber, cucumbers are the perfect ingredient for a healthy summer side dish. Better yet, this cucumber salad is a mere 33 calories per serving.

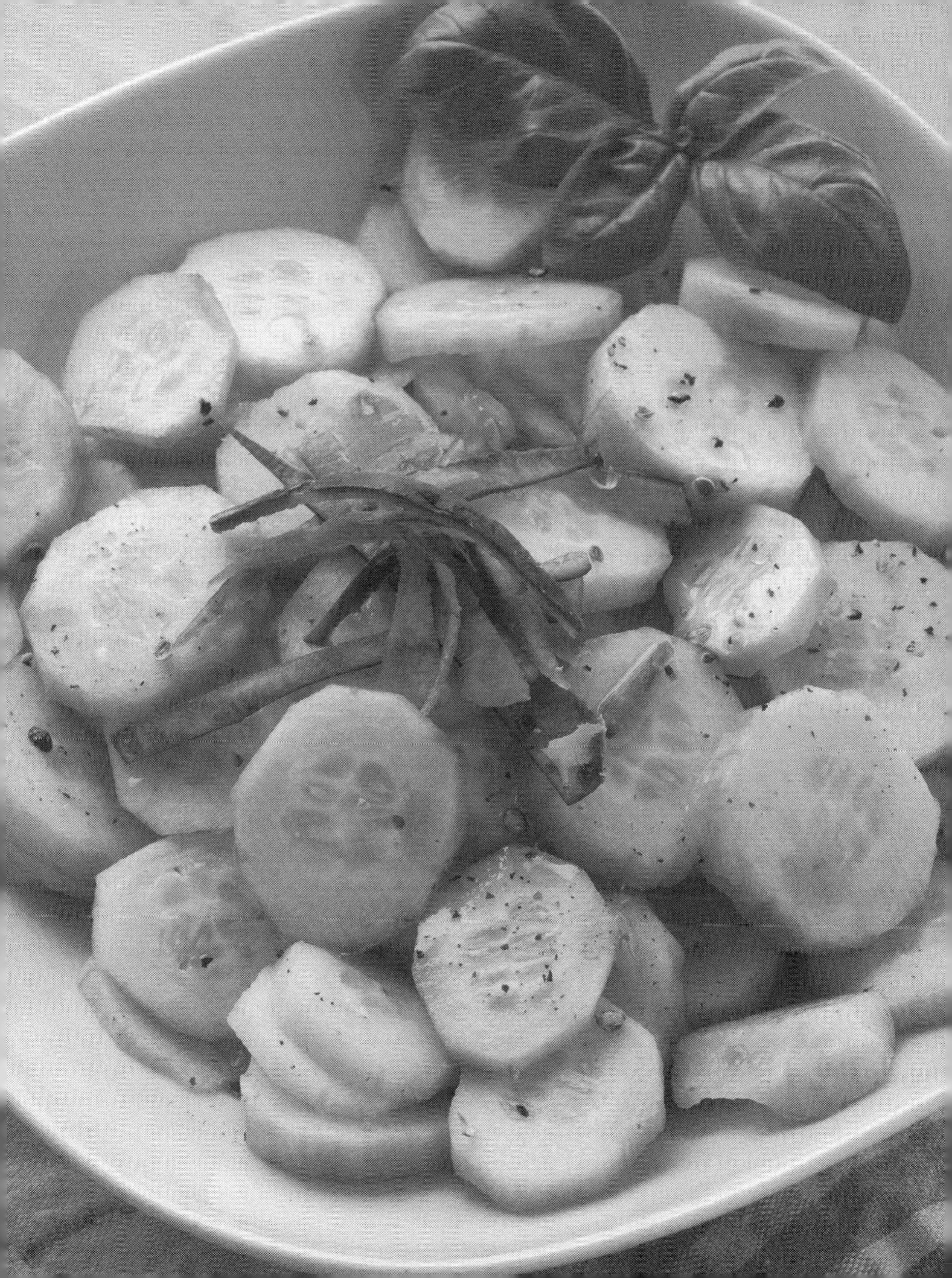

STRAWBERRY SALAD WITH SPINACH AND FETA CHEESE

servings: 6 | calories: 290

Ingredients

- 7 to 10 cups of baby spinach, washed and patted dry
- 5 cups of fresh sliced strawberries
- 1/2 cup of crumbled feta cheese
- 1/4 cup of toasted sliced almonds (optional)
- fat-free dressing of choosing

Directions

1. Toss the baby spinach in a large bowl with the strawberries and toasted almonds, if desired. Mix well and portion into six bowls.
2. Top with the crumbled feta cheese and serve with a dressing of your choice, preferably a low-fat or fat-free variety.
3. Serve immediately. Wrap and refrigerate any leftovers.

Strawberries are considered to be one of the healthiest fruits to eat. Packed with antioxidants and fiber, strawberries can help lower blood pressure and can also protect your heart. They have many nutrients and minerals, are an excellent source of manganese and potassium, and are fat free.

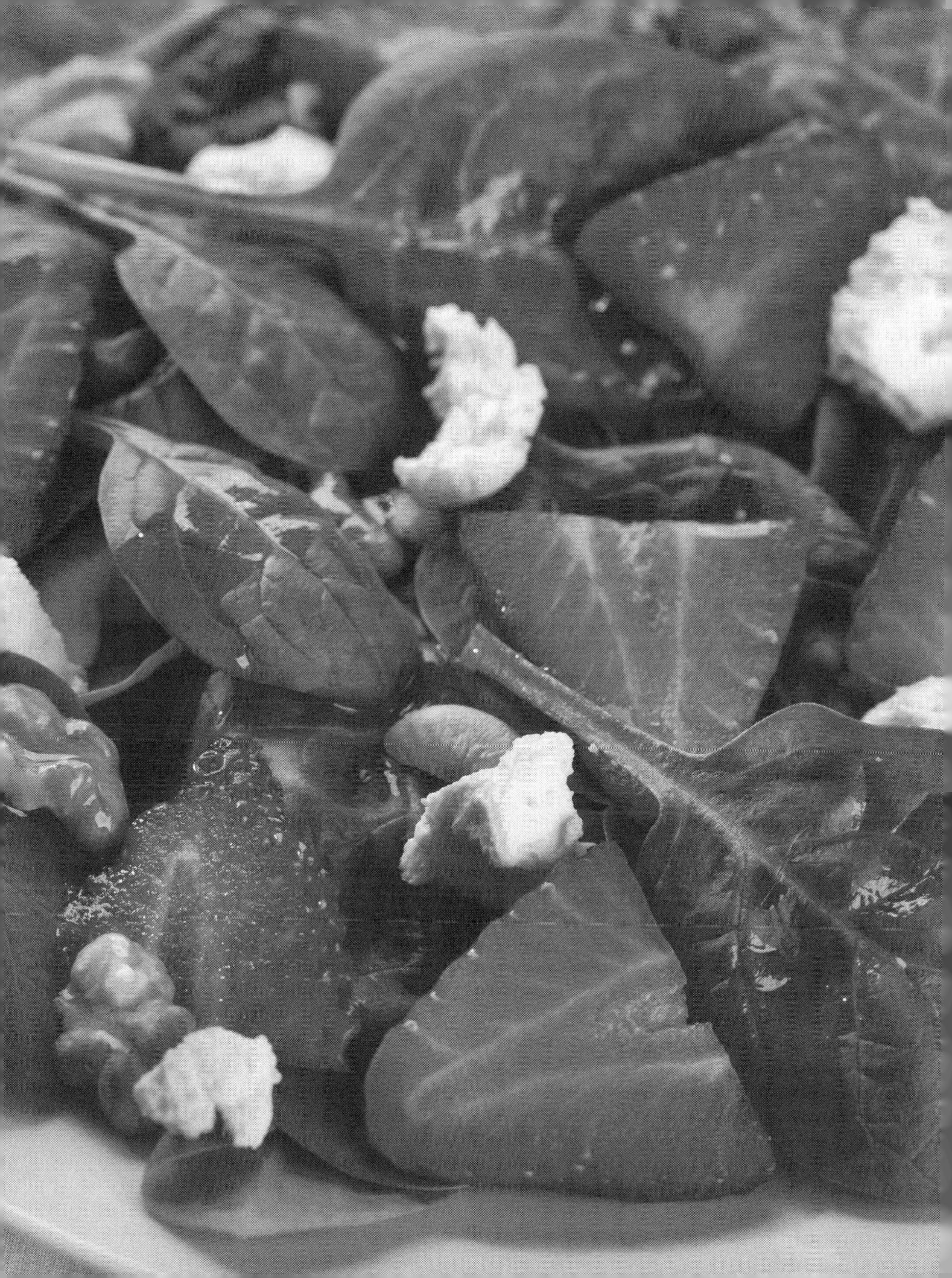

HOMEMADE BACON WRAPPED MUSHROOMS STUFFED WITH CREAM CHEESE

servings: 20 | calories: 123

Ingredients

- 4 cups mushrooms, portobello caps
- 1 1/2 cups cream cheese, softenedr
- 3 tbsps green onions, chopped
- 10 bacon strips

Directions

1. Preheat the oven to 350 degrees Fahrenheit, or 175 degrees Celsius.
2. Mix green onions and cream cheese together in a bowl.
3. Stuff the mushroom caps with the onion and cheese mixture.
4. Cut bacon into half-slices, and wrap around the mushroom caps. Secure with toothpicks to make sure it doesn't fall apart during the cooking process.
5. Spray baking sheet with Pam or some kind of anti-stick cooking spray, and place each bacon-wrapped mushroom cap on the baking sheet.
6. Once the oven has reached 350 degrees Fahrenheit, place the pan inside the oven and bake until the bacon is cooked thoroughly, which usually takes about 20 minutes.

Around our house, bacon is a fan favorite; not only is it tasty, but it's healthy too! But there's no reason you should only have it first thing in the morning. Use this recipe to add a nice side dish to any meal.

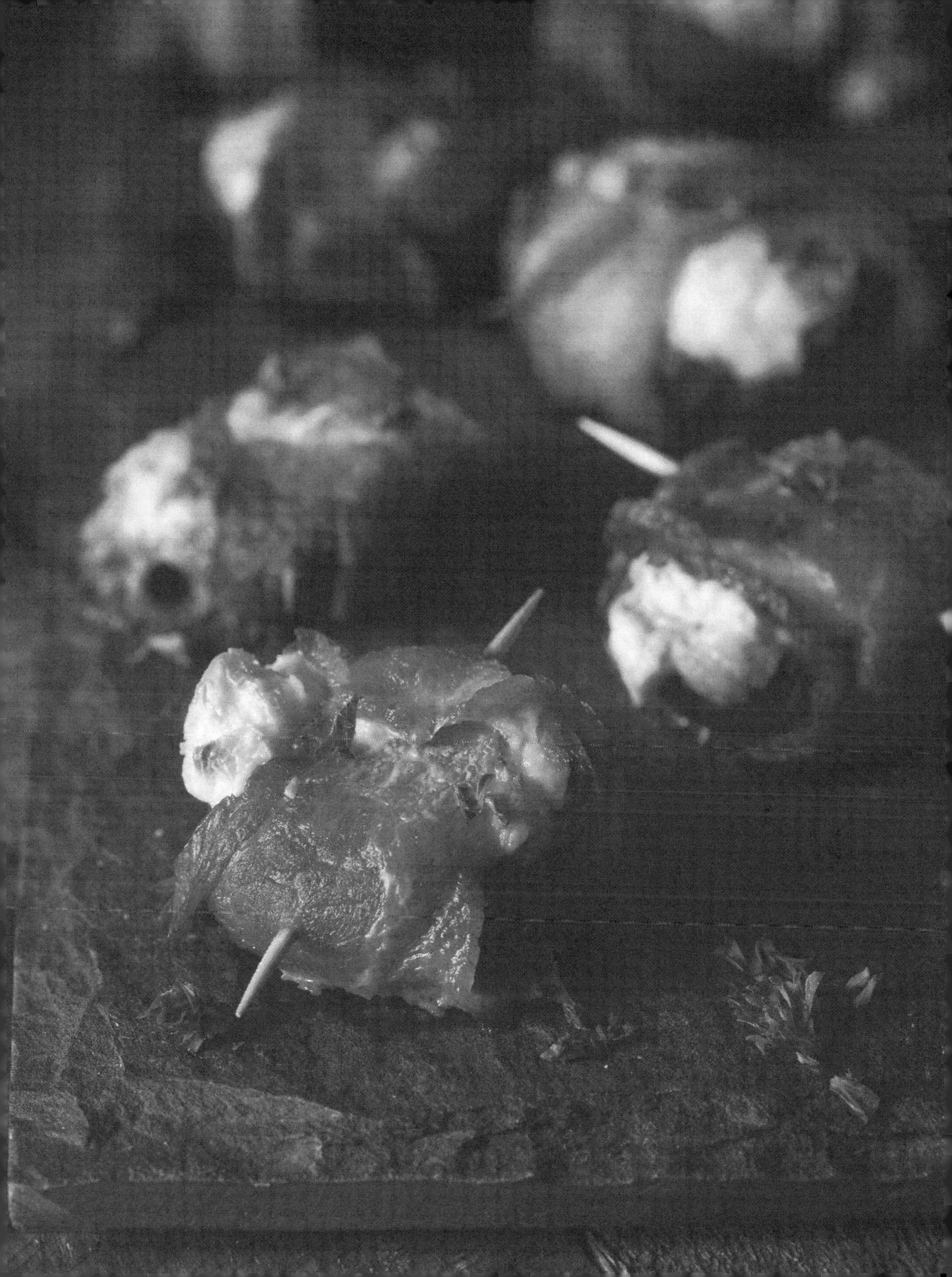

BACON WRAPPED CUTLET WITH GREEN BEANS

servings: 4 | calories: 389

Ingredients

- 8 slices bacon
- 4 skinless, boneless chicken breast halves
- 4 cups green beans
- 6 ounces cream cheese, softened
- green onions, chopped
- 1/4 cup chopped red bell pepper
- 1 tsp garlic powder
- 1 tsp salt
- 1/2 tsp pepper

Directions

1. Preheat the oven to 350 degrees Fahrenheit, or 175 degrees Celsius.
2. Mix together the cream cheese, green onions, bell pepper, garlic powder, salt, and pepper in a bowl until combined. Divide this mixture onto each chicken breast. Fold the breasts in half, and wrap with 2 slices of bacon. Secure with toothpicks to make sure it doesn't fall apart during the cooking process.
3. Spray baking sheet with some kind of cooking spray, and place each bacon-wrapped cutlets on the baking sheet.
4. Once the oven has reached 350 degrees Fahrenheit, place the pan inside the oven and bake for about 30 - 35 minutes until thickest part of chicken is no longer pink.
5. Steam the green beans to desired texture, 5 - 10 minutes and serve with the bacon wrapped cutlets.

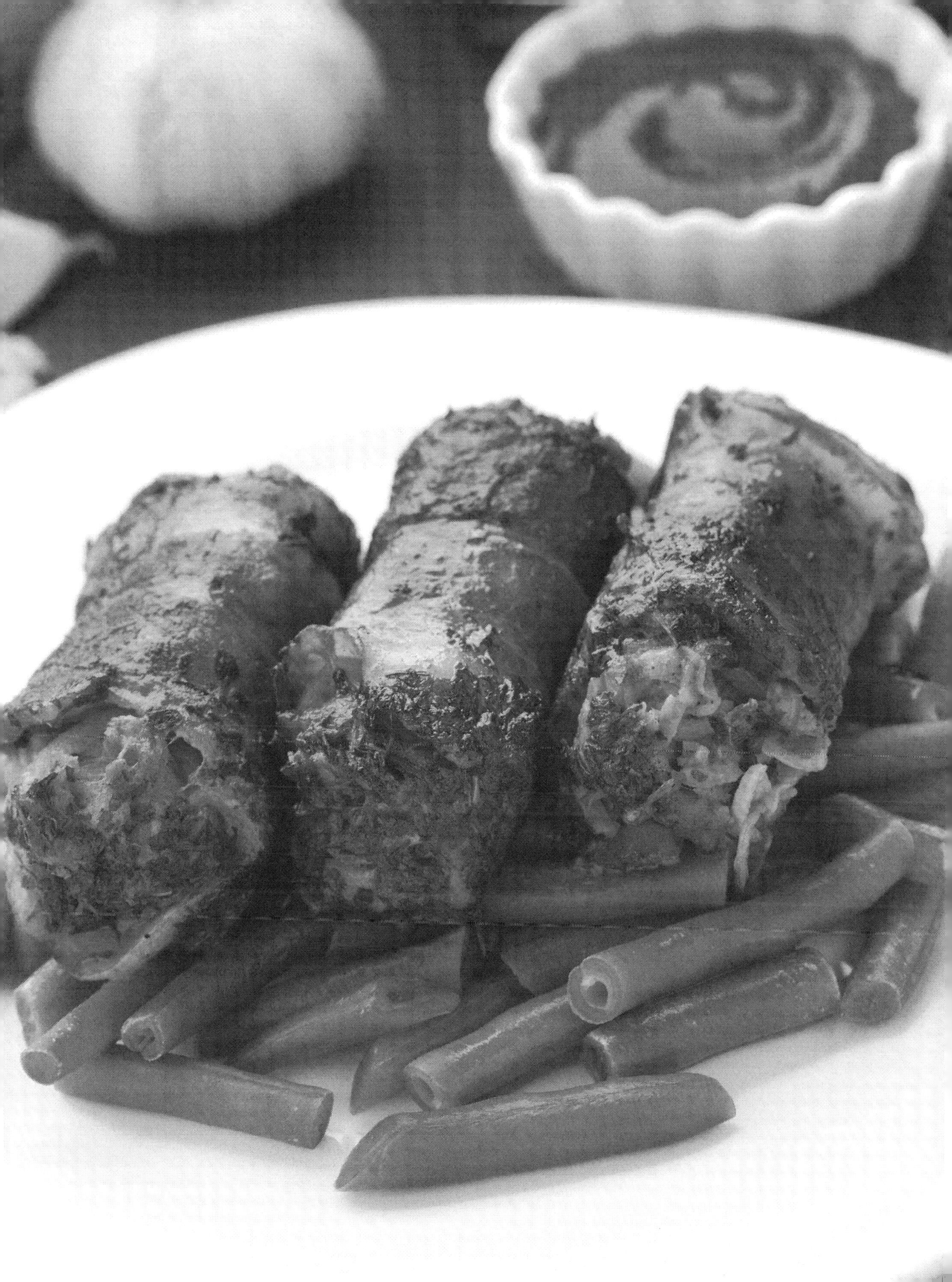

BACON WRAPPED CHICKEN THIGH STUFFED WITH WINE SAUCE AND BRUSSEL SPROUTS

servings: 6 | calories: 216

Ingredients

- 6 chicken thighs (skinless and deboned)
- 1 package of bacon (about 12 pieces)
- 2 cups of brussel sprouts
- 1 table spoon of olive oil

White Wine Sauce

- 1/3 cup of chopped onion
- 1 chicken stock cube
- 1/2 cup of white wine
- 2 table spoons of butter

Directions

1. In a medium sauce pan, combine ingredients for white wine sauce and warm over medium heat for five minutes. Reduce heat and allow sauce to thicken as it cools.
2. Cut skinless, deboned, chicken thighs into small cubes. Add olive oil to a medium skillet and brown chicken thighs on both sides for 1-2 minutes. Remove chicken from pan and set aside.
3. Wrap each chicken thigh cube in 1 strip of bacon. Fill a medium casserole dish with white wine sauce and add chicken thighs. Bake for 30 minutes at 350 degrees.

Bacon wrapped chicken thighs stuffed with wine sauce and brussel sprouts is a dish that combines protein rich chicken with beneficial brussel sprouts that are filled with vitamins C and K. This dish combines helpful nutrient-dense foods with the flavorful addition of bacon and wine sauce to create an impactful meal.

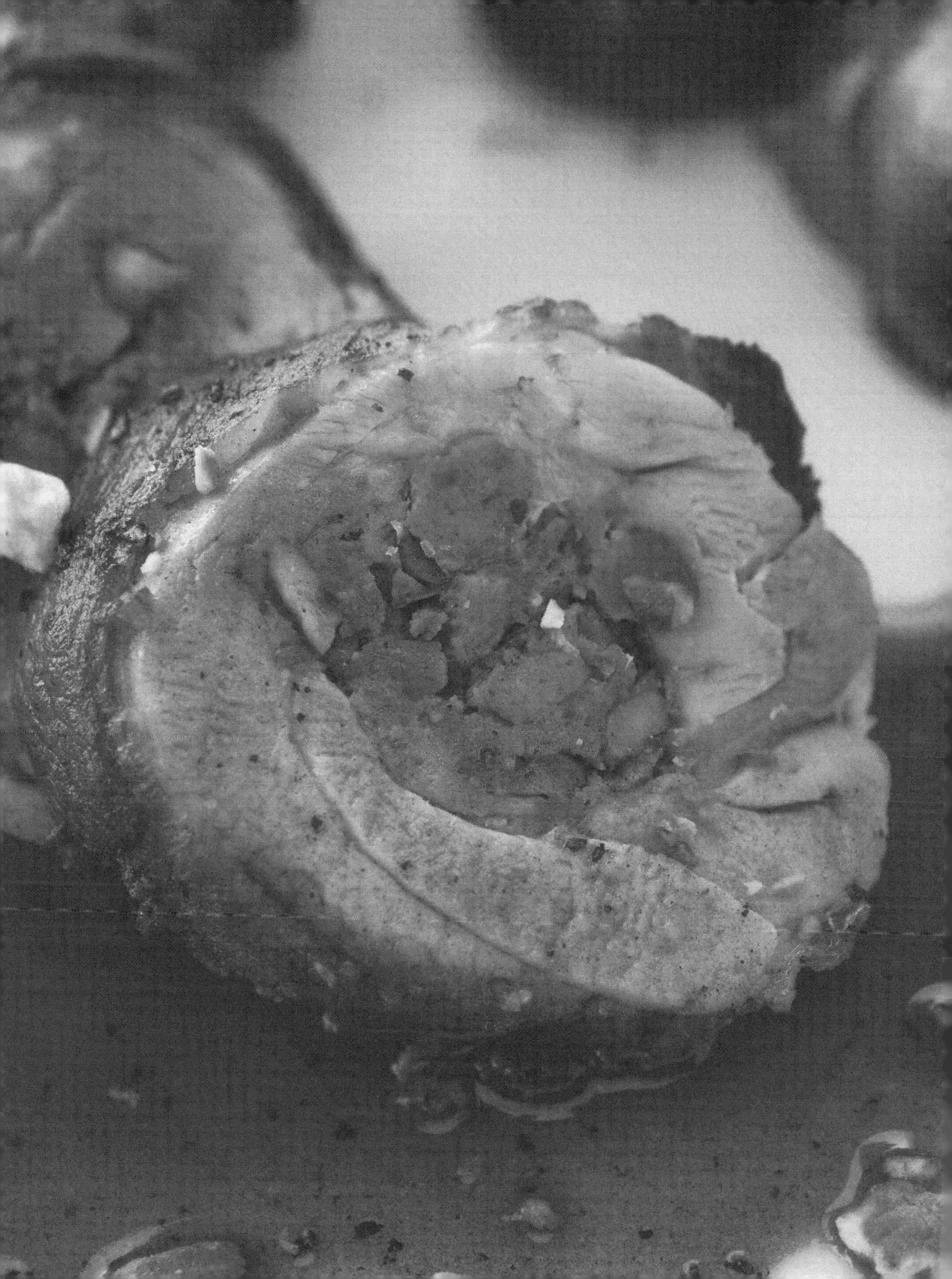

GRILLED ATLANTIC SALMON WITH A ROCKET SALAD, CAPERS, PARSLEY AND LEMON

servings: 4

Ingredients

For The Salmon:

4 atlantic salmon filets

1 tbsp extra virgin olive oil

2 tbsps lemon juice

salt, to taste

pepper, to taste

1 tsp garlic powder

For The Salad:

1 lb rocket arugula

1/2 cup fresh, chopped parsley

1 tbsp extra virgin olive oil

1 - 2 tbsps lemon juice, to taste

salt and pepper, to taste

2 tbsps caper berries, roughly chopped

Directions

1. Preheat the grill to 350 degrees Fahrenheit.
2. Leave the skin on the salmon filets. Brush the salmon filets with olive oil on both sides. Place the salmon filets skin side down on the grill. Drizzle lemon juice on the flesh and then sprinkle with garlic powder, salt, and pepper. Grill until cooked all the way through. This should take about 15 minutes.
3. While the salmon is grilling, prepare the salad. Toss the rocket (arugula) into a mixing bowl. Add the parsley, olive oil, lemon juice, salt, and pepper. Toss with a pair of salad tongs until the ingredients are well coated. Top with capers.
4. Distribute the salad evenly between four plates. Top each bed of arugula with a cooked salmon filet. Serve immediately.

Salmon is rich in Omega 3 fatty acids and is also high in protein. The salad is packed with nutrients. Rocket, also known as arugula, is a great source of Vitamin A, Vitamin K, Vitamin C, and also folate. Parsley is also a nutrient powerhouse and is rich in vitamins and minerals such as Vitamin A, Vitamin C, Vitamin K, Vitamin E, and Potassium.

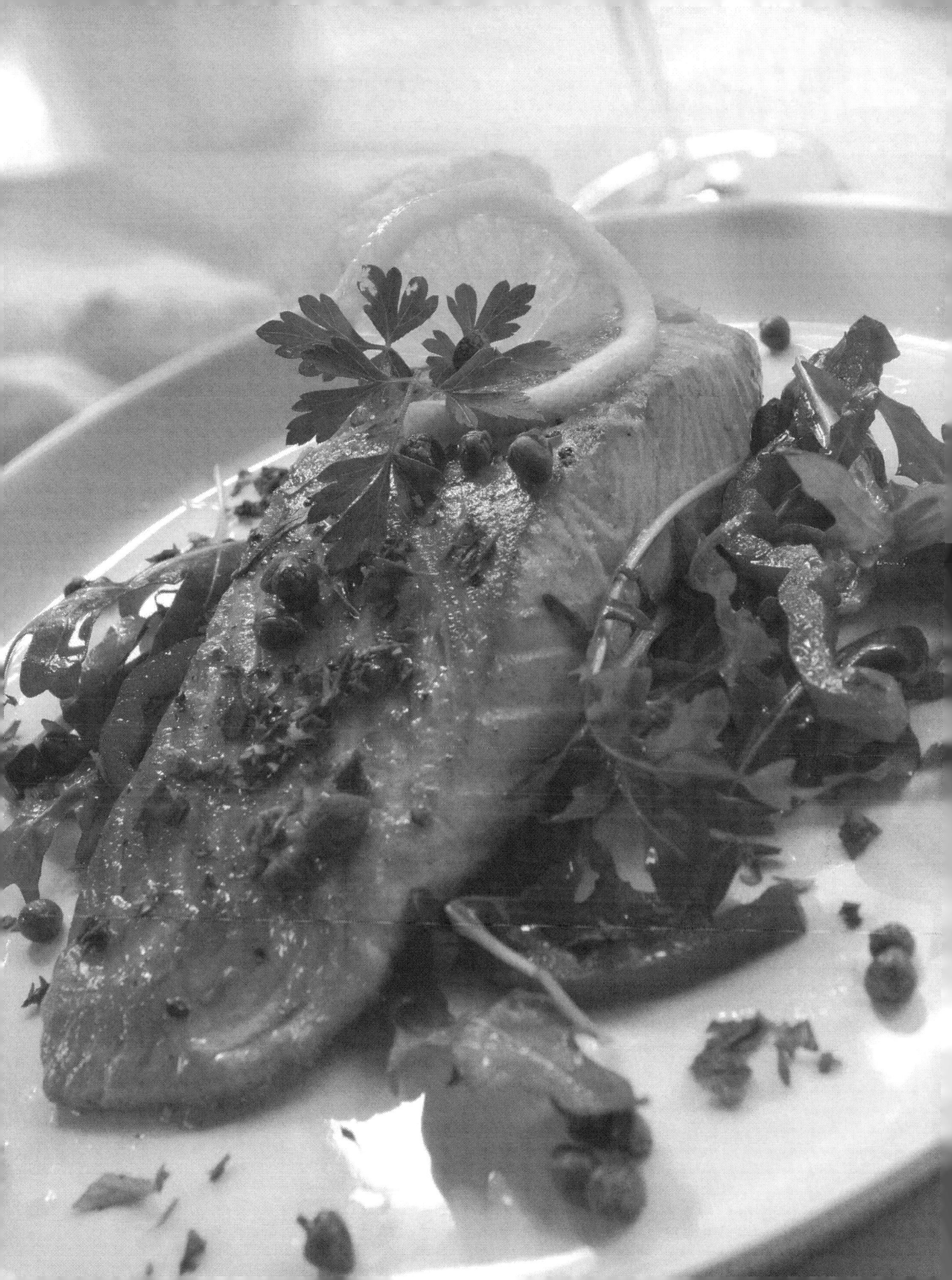

SEARED TUNA NICOISE SALAD

servings: 6 | calories: 350

Ingredients

- 1 lb fresh tuna
- 3/4 lb red boiled potatoes
- 1 1/2 tbsp red wine vinegar
- 5 chopped garlic cloves
- 7 tbsp olive oil
- 1 1/2 tbsp dijon mustard
- 1 1/2 cups water
- 1 yellow pepper
- 3/4 lb string beans
- 1 1/2 cups red onion, sliced
- 1 cup nicoise olives
- 1 dozen red lettuce leaves
- 1 tsp canola oil
- 1 cup shredded basil
- 3 tsp black pepper
- 2 tsp salt

Directions

1. Dressing is prepared in large bowl by whisking vinegar, garlic, mustard, 1 tsp salt and pepper, and olive oil. Peep potatoes and cut into slices measuring 1/2 inch, toss with dressing.
2. Boil green beans in water, drain, and cut in half. Cut peeled yellow pepper into julienne strips. Cut tomatoes in half and de-seed. Add peppers, beans, tomatoes, black olives, and red peppers to the potato and dressing mix and combine.
3. Once you're nearly ready to serve, sear fresh tuna in cast-iron or heavy skillet on high heat for 2 minutes on each side with canola oil and remaining salt/pepper. Saute on either side another 2 minutes.
4. Cut into 1/2 inch slices and serve atop salad with basil and red lettuce leaves.

A fresh source of lean protein and omega-3 fatty acids, this tuna salad recipe yields 6 servings.

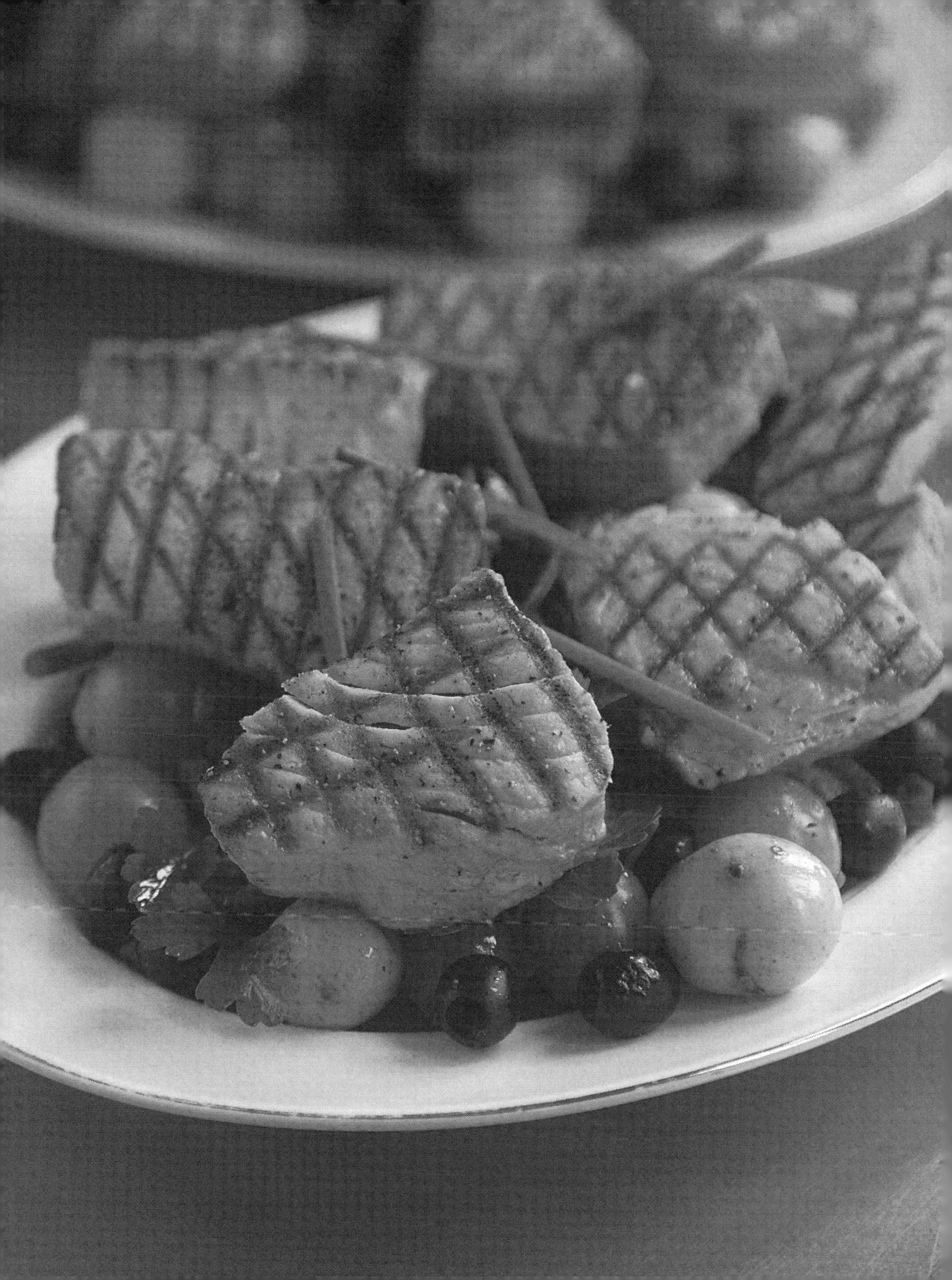

SEARED AHI TUNA COATED WITH SESAME SEEDS AND GREEN SALAD

servings: 4 | calories: 200

Ingredients

- 1 lb fresh tuna
- 1 tbsp of oil
- 2 tbsps white sesame seeds
- 2 tbsps black sesame seeds
- 1 large sliced avocado
- 1 cup of sliced cucumbers
- 1/2 cup julienned carrots
- 1/2 cup edamame
- 2 sliced green onions
- 2 tbsps pickled ginger.

Directions

1. To prepare the tuna, heat one tablespoon of oil over medium-high heat.
2. Press two tablespoons of white sesame seeds and two tablespoons of black sesame seeds into the tuna on all sides. Sear the tuna for one or two minutes on each side. Let cool for a few minutes and slice.
3. For the salad, start with six cups of salad greens.
4. Add one large sliced avocado, one cup of sliced cucumbers, half a cup of julienned carrots, half a cup of edamame, two sliced green onions, and two tablespoons of pickled ginger.
5. Toss everything with your favorite dressing and enjoy!

Tuna is an excellent source of protein and is full of omega-3 fatty acids and magnesium. Try seared ahi tuna to bring out the delicious flavor and serve with fresh greens for additional nutrients and a savory healthy meal.

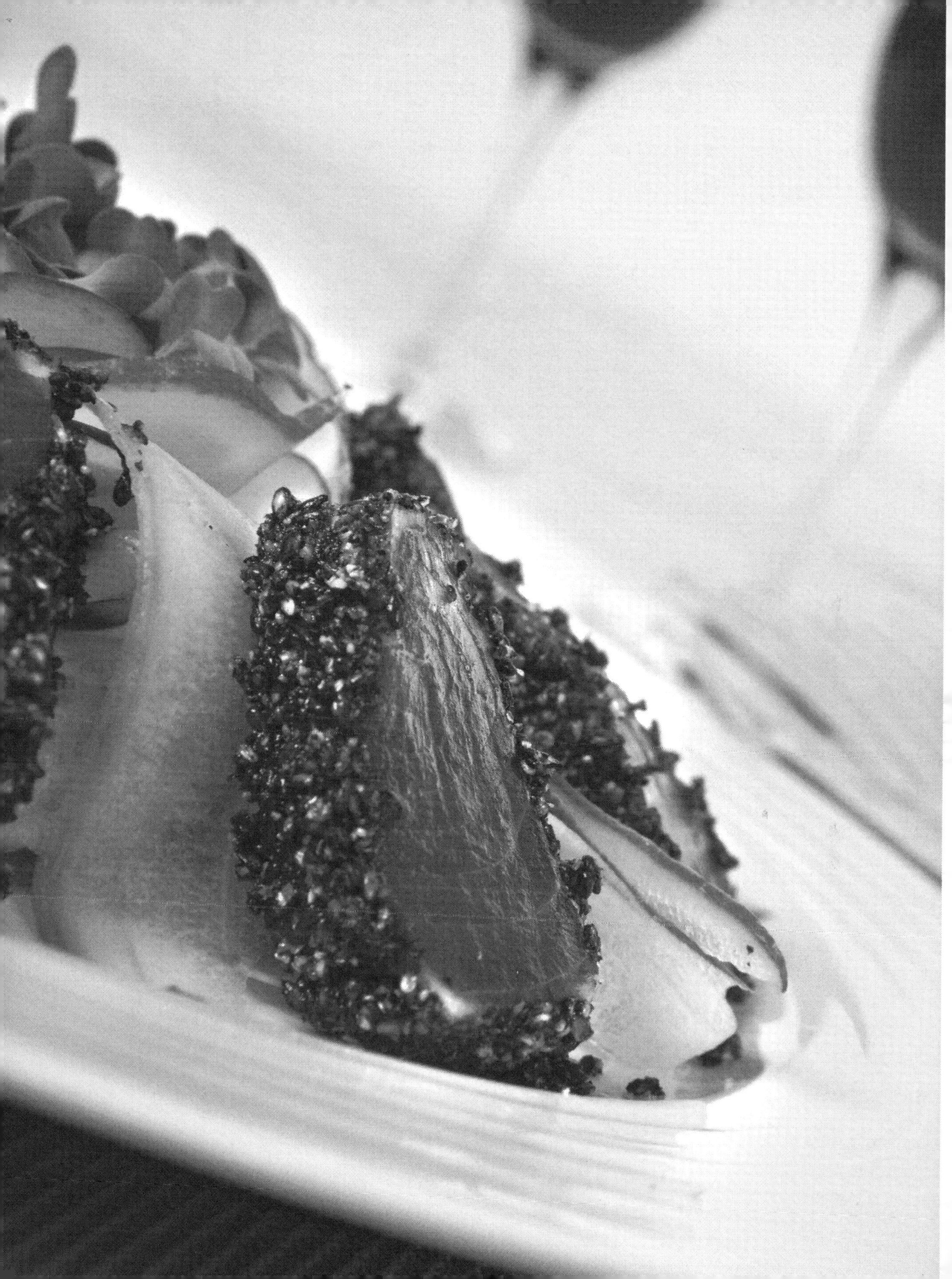

SWEET LEMON SHRIMP

servings: 4 | calories: 500

Ingredients

- 1 1/2 lbs of peeled shrimp
- 1/2 cup fresh squeezed lemon juice
- 1/4 cup soy sauce
- 1/4 cup honey
- 1 lemon, zest
- 2 tbsps chopped cilantro
- salt and pepper to taste

Directions

1. Begin by placing the honey, pepper, salt, soy sauce, lemon juice, lemon zest in a medium bowl.
2. In another bowl, combine the mixture from the medium bowl with the shrimp. Allow the ingredients to marinate for about 30 minutes. If possible, leave marinating overnight. Make sure to turn the bag.
3. Preheat oven to 400 degrees F.
4. Use aluminum foil to line the baking sheet.
5. Discard marinate and place shrimp on baking sheet.
6. Place into oven and cook for about 6-8 minutes.
7. Use cilantro as garnish.

Shrimp is low-fat, contains Omega-3 fatty acids and is a good source of vitamin B12 and vitamin D.

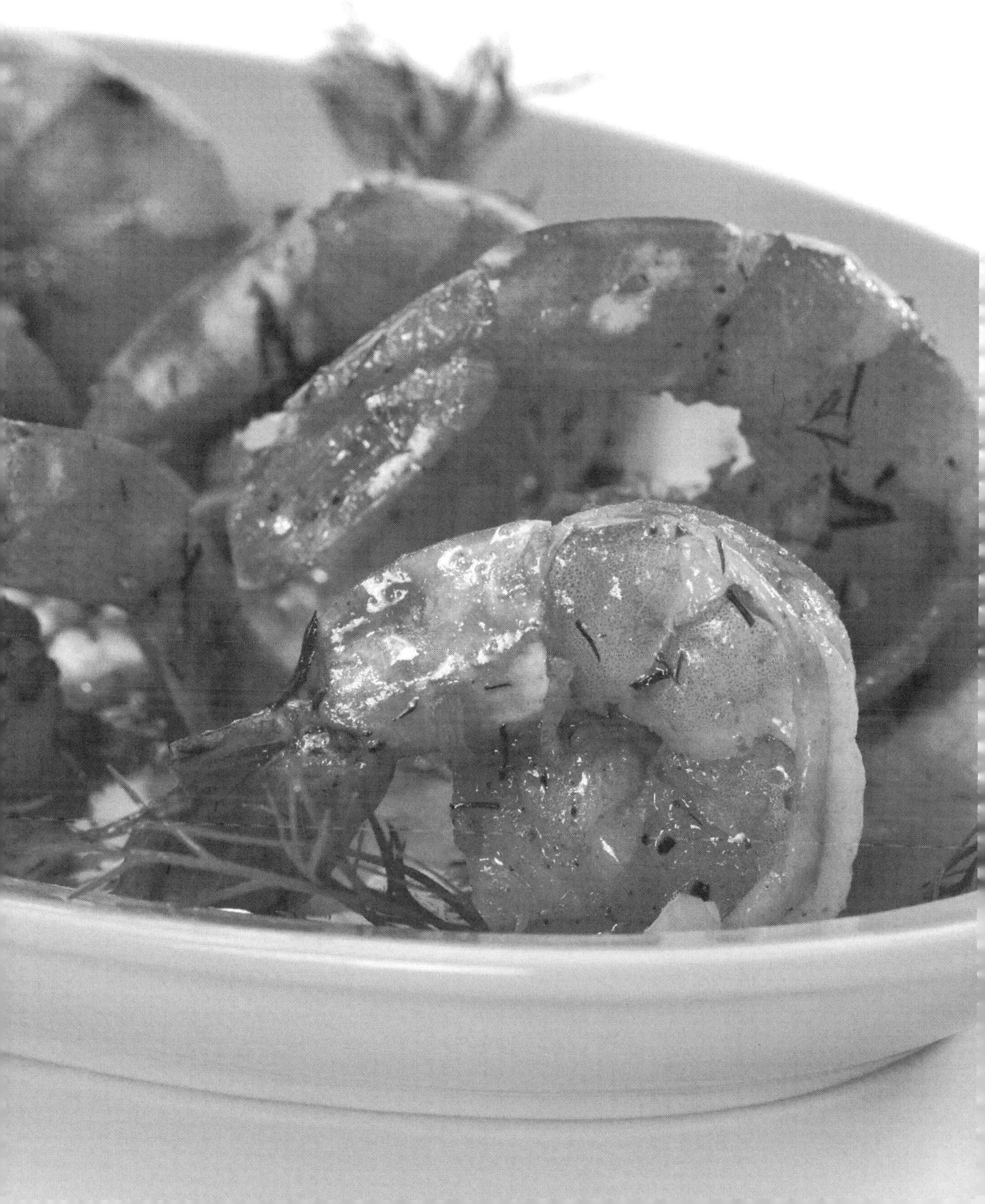

BACON WRAPPED SHRIMP

servings: 4 - 6 | calories: 110

Ingredients

- 16 large fresh, peeled and deveined shrimp
- 8 slices of bacon, uncooked
- BBQ seasoning to taste

Directions

1. Preheat oven to 450 degrees.
2. Wrap each shrimp with ½ slice of bacon and secure with a toothpick to keep bacon on.
3. Line a baking sheet with foil and place wrapped shrimp an inch apart from one another. Sprinkle with a small amount of BBQ seasoning to taste.
4. Cook for 10 to 15 minutes or until the bacon is done. Turn the wrap if needed.

Bacon wrapped shrimp is not just a yummy meal, it can be good for you, too! Shrimp is a great source of vitamin B12, copper, iodine, protein and selenium, which are nutrients we may be lacking.

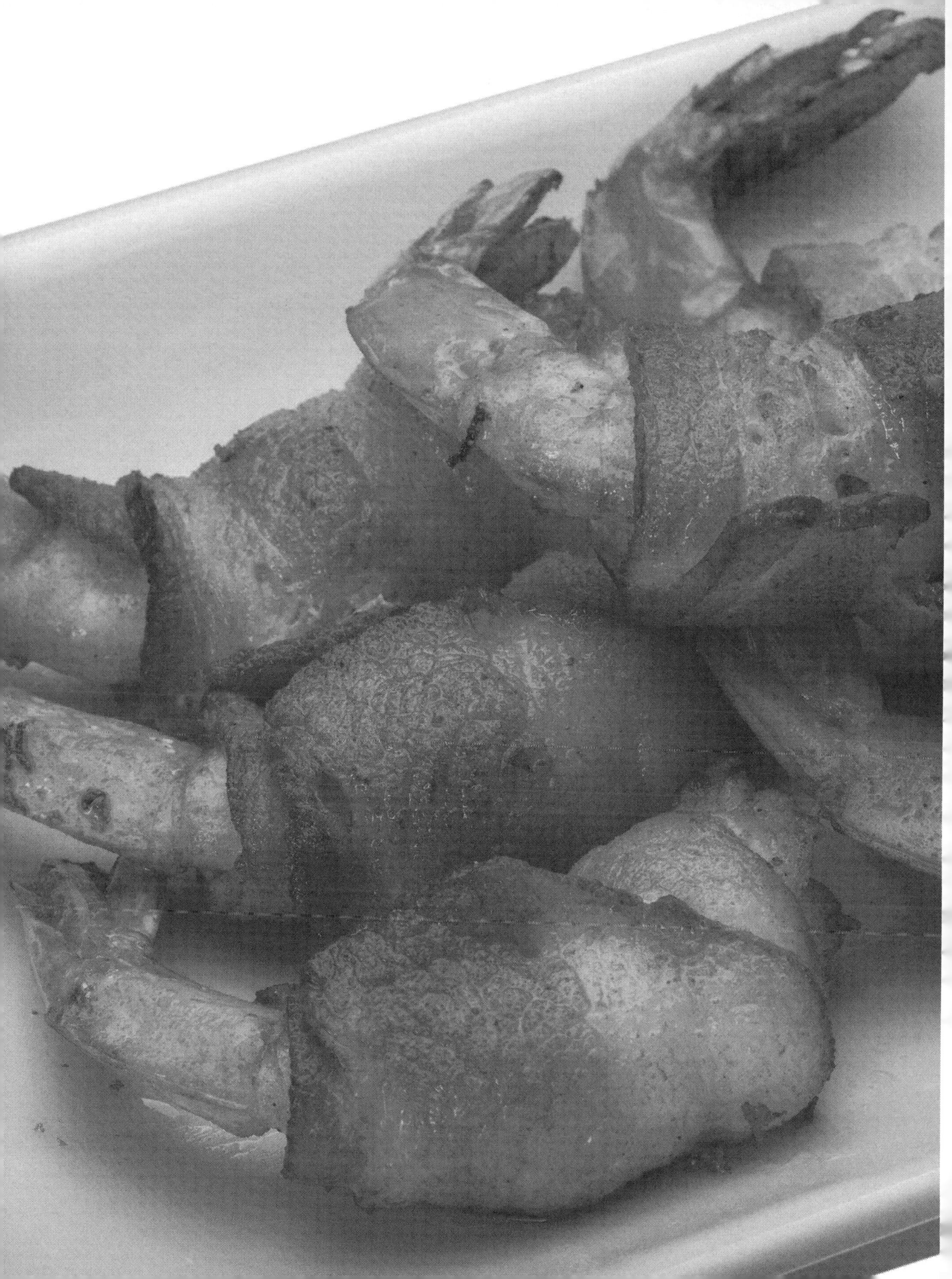

MUSSELS WITH WHITE WINE SAUCE

servings: 4 | calories: 238

Ingredients

- 1 tablespoon olive oil
- 3 garlic cloves (minced)
- 1/8 teaspoon red pepper flakes (or to taste)
- 1 cup white wine
- 3 sprigs of thyme (fresh)
- 2 bay leaves, whole
- 4 lbs mussels, scrubbed & debearded
- 1/4 teaspoon salt
- 2 tablespoons butter (cut into 4 pieces)
- 2 tablespoons parsley (freshly minced)

Directions

1. Heat the oven to 500 degrees with the oven rack in the lowest position--close to the heating element.
2. Begin by using the roasting pan directly on the stove top. Heat the pan over medium heat with the garlic, oil, and red pepper flakes for 30 seconds.
3. Once the oil is fragrant and garlic is straw colored, add wine, thyme, and bay leaves. The mixture should boil for about a minute.
4. Add the cleaned mussels with salt to the roasting pan. Cover tightly with foil and place in the oven. After 15-18 minutes peek under the foil to see if the majority of the mussels have opened. If so, remove from oven.
5. With mussels pushed to the side of the pan, add butter to the juices in the pan--whisking it in. Spoon the buttery sauce on top of the mussels and sprinkle with parsley.
6. Serve immediately over cooked pasta or dip a baguette into the sauce.

The natural antioxidant benefits of wine and the burst of omega-3 fatty acids from mussels pack a 1-2 punch to your body. A dish that's sophisticated and health conscious--Mussels with White Wine Sauce is the perfect meal that is sure to impress.

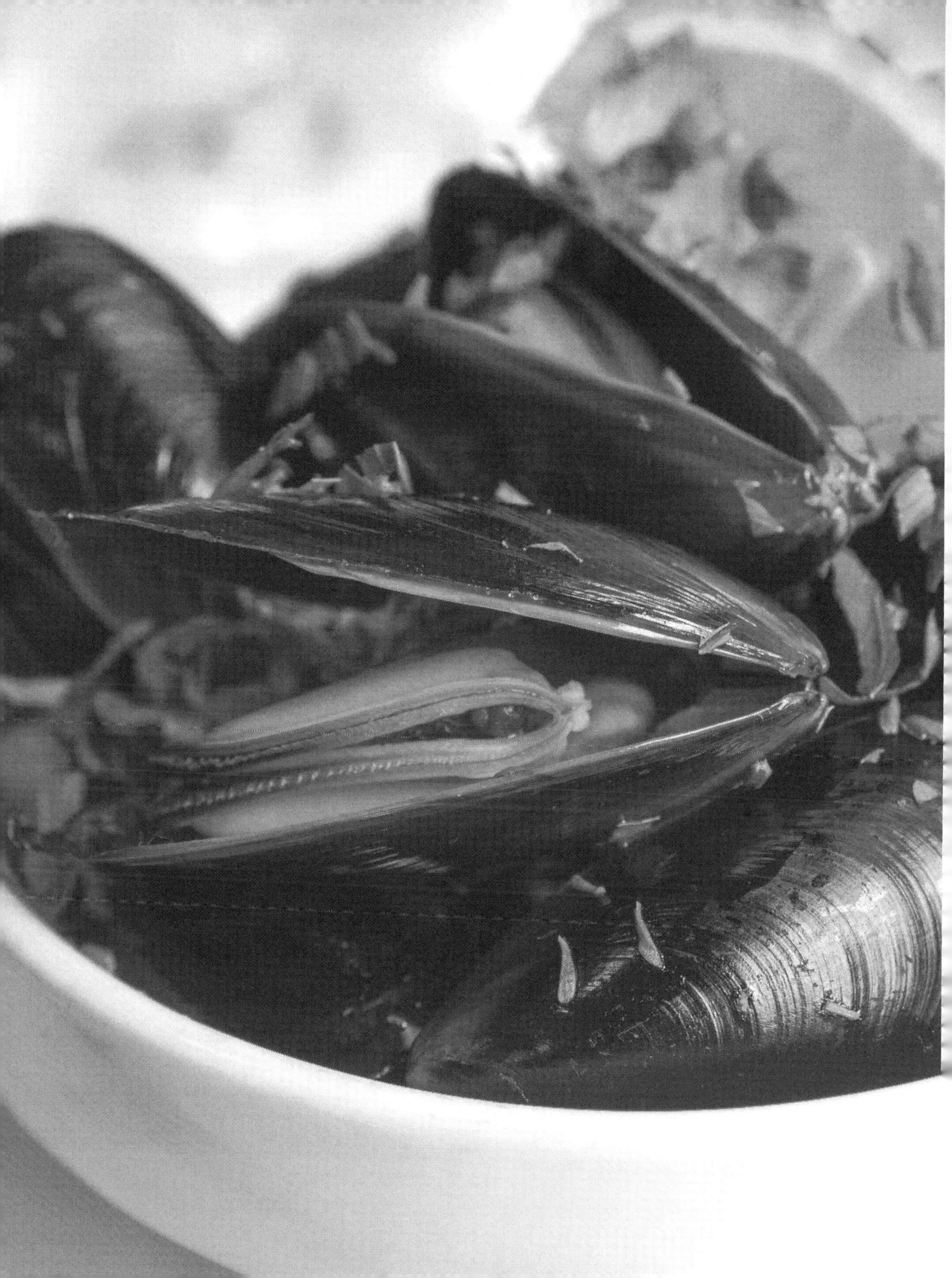

SHRIMP WITH WHITE WINE SAUCE

servings: 4 - 5 | calories: 290

Ingredients

- 12 large, peeled/deveined shrimp
- 1 lemon
- 1/2 cup white wine
- 4 garlic cloves, finely chopped
- 1/4 cup olive oil
- 1 cup finely chopped parsley
- 1 tbsp butter, cubed
- black pepper to taste
- 1/4 tsp red pepper flakes - optional for spice

Directions

1. On med-high heat, heat up the oil and add shrimp. Saute for no longer than one minute. Add in garlic and flip shrimp for the same amount of time on other side. Cook on either side twice more for the same amount of time. Pour in wine and cover. Let it simmer for one minute. Remove lid.
2. Continue to cook the wine sauce, adding in the butter, pepper, parsley, pepper flakes, and lemon juice.
3. Serve over angel hair pasta or linguine.

Shrimp provides a lean source of healthy protein.

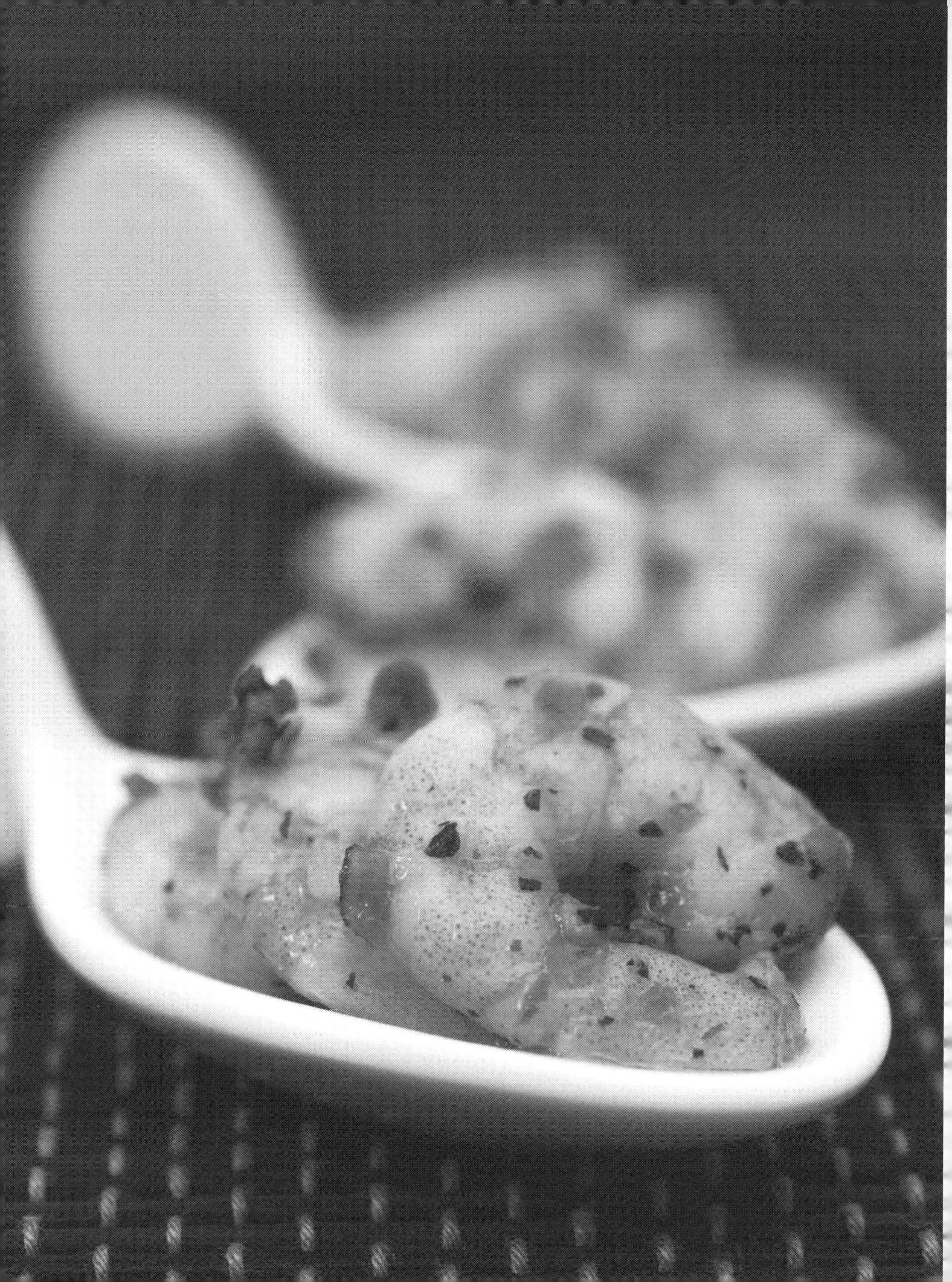

PULLED PORK AND FRIED POTATOES

servings: 6 | calories: 637

Ingredients

- 1 10 ounces bone-in pork butt
- 2 tsps of ground coriander
- 1 tsp of toasted ground cumin
- 1/2 tsp of garlic powder
- 2 tbsps Kosher salt
- 2 tsps of cracked black pepper

Directions

1. Pulled pork with fried potatoes is a favorite of many cooks, creating a dish that is high in protein and carbs, without excess trans fat.
2. Combine 2 tablespoons Kosher salt with 2 teaspoons of cracked black pepper, 2 teaspoons of ground coriander, 1 teaspoon of toasted ground cumin, and 1/2 teaspoon of garlic powder, rubbing the mixture into 1 bone-in pork butt.
3. Place pork butt in smoker at 225 degrees Fahrenheit, and smoke for 6-8 hours or until internal temperature is 195 degrees Fahrenheit. Let sit for 30 minutes, and shred with a fork, mixing with BBQ sauce.
4. Create the BBQ sauce by combining vinegar, red onion, garlic, chipotle, bourbon, coriander, paprika, and horseradish, bringing it to a boil and then reducing to a simmer for ten minutes. Strain in a mixing bowl, and add in stadium mustard, yellow mustard, maple syrup, soy sauce, kosher salt, and cracked black pepper.
5. Add garlic, herbs and whole potatoes to a boil in salted water until potatoes are tender. Drain, and break potatoes apart. Heat canola oil to 375 degrees Fahrenheit, frying potatoes until crunchy.
6. To serve, place potatoes on a platter, top with pork, BBQ sauce, and enjoy.

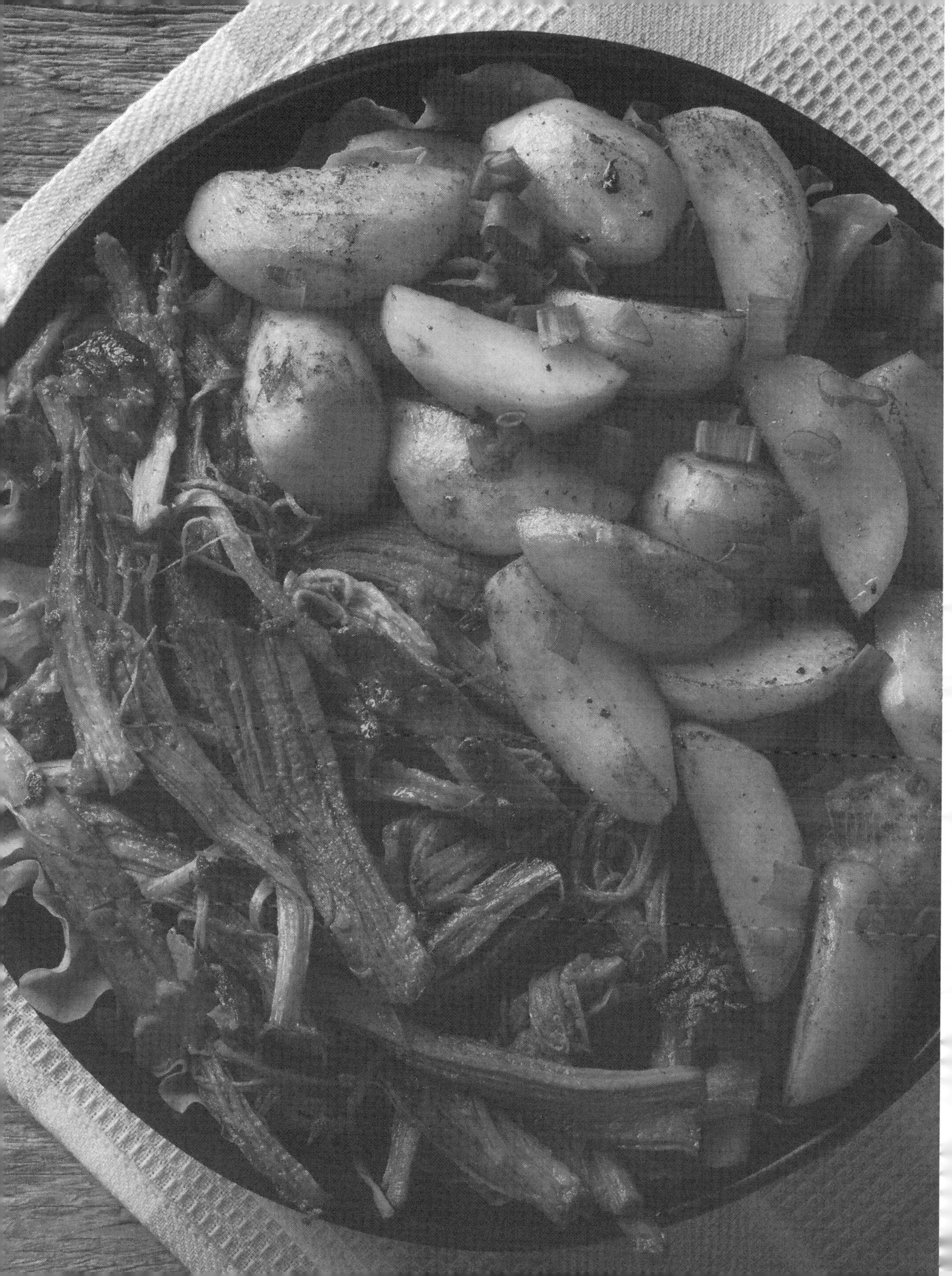

LOBSTER WITH GARLIC AND SPRING ONIONS

servings: 4 | calories: 132

Ingredients

- 4 - 3 oz lobster tails
- 1/2 cup spring onions, chopped
- 1 cup chicken broth
- 2 tsps garlic, minced
- 2 tbsps ginger, minced
- 2 tbsps fish sauce
- 1 tbsp rice vinegar
- 2 tbsps sesame oil

Directions

1. Separate lobster meat from shell. Cube lobster meat and set aside. Saute onions and ginger in sesame oil until onions are clear and tender.
2. Add lobster and saute for five minutes. Add remaining ingredients. Reduce heat, simmer for seven minutes.
3. Serve over noodles or rice.

This meal proves healthy and delicious can coexist. High in protein, low in carbs, and with less than four grams of fat per serving, Lobster with spring onions is also bursting with flavor, since spring onions are more flavorful than regular onions. This meal is delicious and very easy to make, taking less than one hour to prepare and cook.

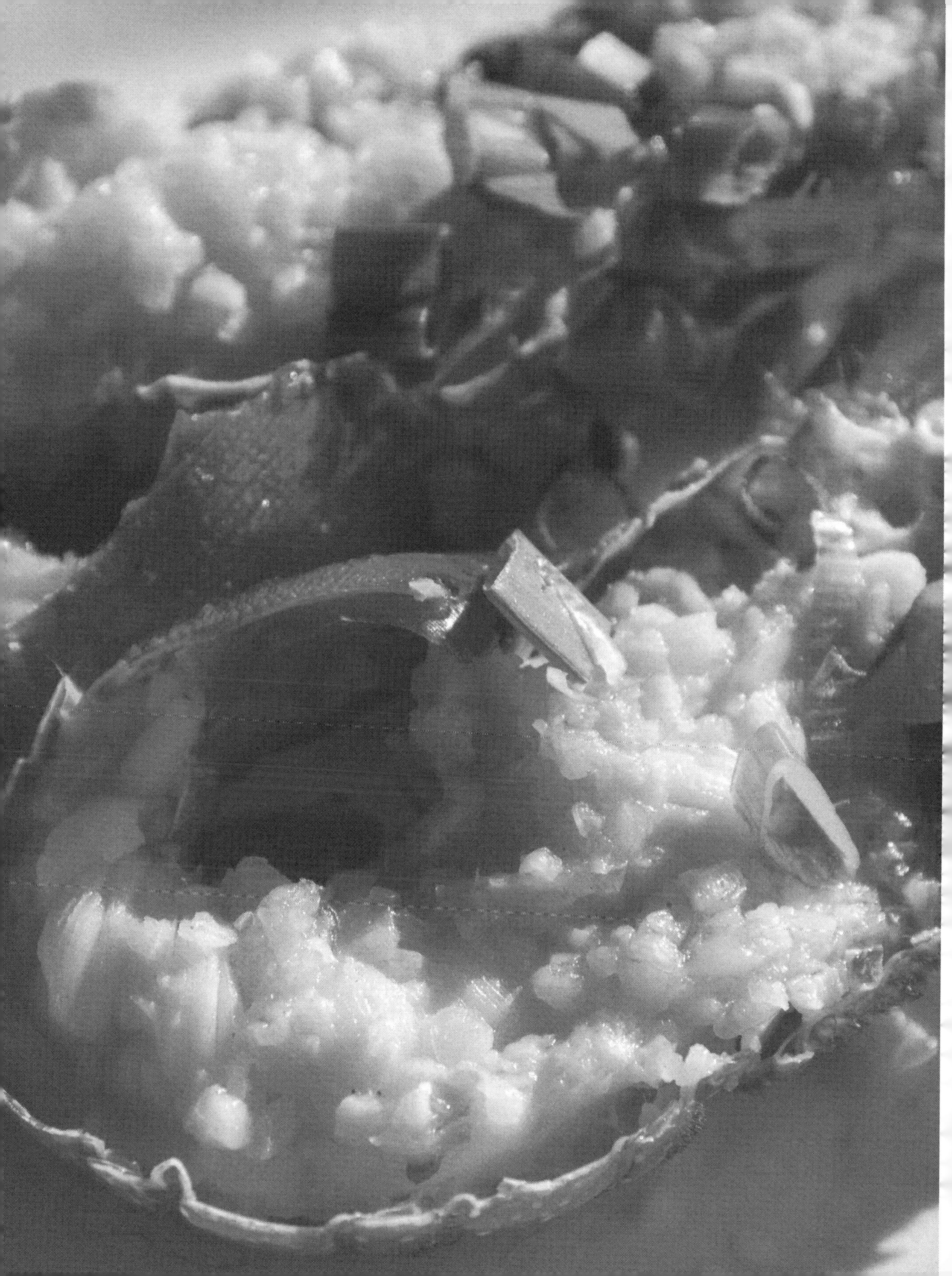

PRAWN IN SWEET AND SPICY SAUCE

servings: 4 - 6 | calories: 250

Ingredients

- 12 prawns, peeled and deveined
- 2 tsps of cornstarch
- 1 tbsp of soy sauce
- 1 tbsp of honey
- 1 tbsp of cider vinegar
- 1 1/2 tsps of chili garlic sauce
- 1 tbsp vegetable oil
- 2 garlic cloves, chopped
- 1 tsp fresh ginger grated
- 1 shallot, finely chopped
- 1/2 tsp of salt
- 1/4 tsp of ground pepper.

Directions

1. Add them to a large bowl with two teaspoons of cornstarch, 1/2 teaspoon of salt, and 1/4 teaspoon of ground pepper.
2. Prepare the sauce in a separate bowl. Mix one tablespoon of soy sauce, one tablespoon of honey, one tablespoon of cider vinegar, and one and a half teaspoons of chili garlic sauce.
3. Next, add one tablespoon of vegetable oil to a large skillet, over high heat. Add two cloves of chopped garlic, one teaspoon of grated fresh ginger, and one finely chopped shallot.
4. Add the prawns and stir fry for two minutes. Coat the prawns with the sauce. Enjoy!

Prawns are a great source of protein, but still low in fat, making them a delicious and healthy idea for dinner. A sweet and spicy sauce gives them a unique taste that can satisfy any craving.

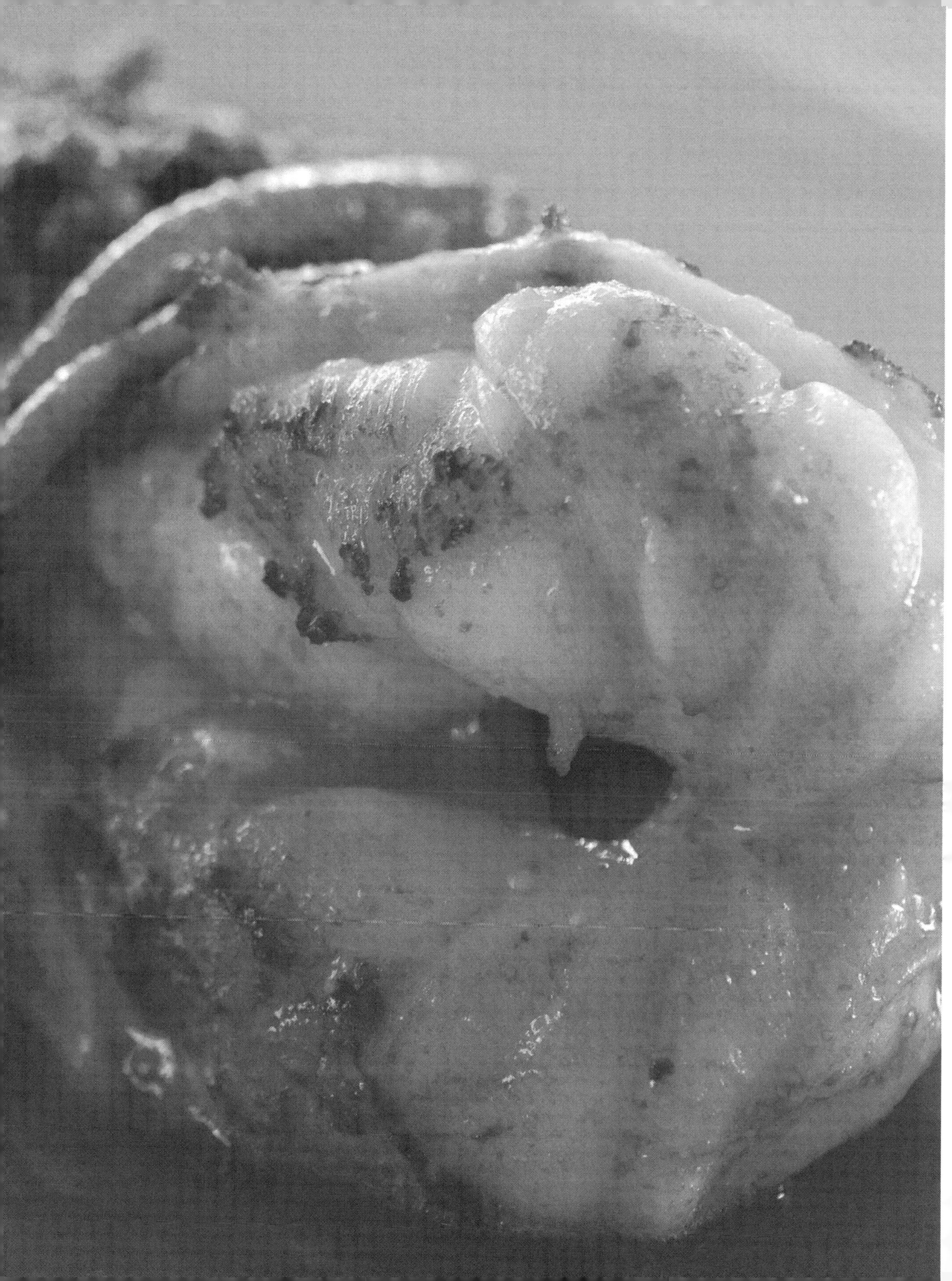

STIR FRIED SHRIMPS WITH HERBS

servings: 4 - 6 | calories: 888

Ingredients

- 1 lb jumbo shrimp (peeled and deveined)
- 1 lb of egg noodles(uncooked)
- 12-16 ounces of frozen peas
- 1/2 tsp dried thyme
- 1 bunch of leek
- lemon
- 4 tsps fresh chives
- 1/2 cup butter

Directions

1. Combine the butter, chives, and lemon peel in a bowl. Once combined melt over medium heat. Proceed to add they thyme and leeks to the herb butter. Begin to cook the noodles in a separate pan.
2. While the noodles cook, add shrimp and lemon juice to herb butter. Stir fry for 6 minutes. Once complete add the noodles to the herb butter mixture.
3. Serve immediately.

This stir fried shrimp with herbs recipe is a dish that you and your family will love. With the high levels of B vitamins and trace metals found in shrimp, you can rest assured knowing that you are making a delicious but nutritious meal.

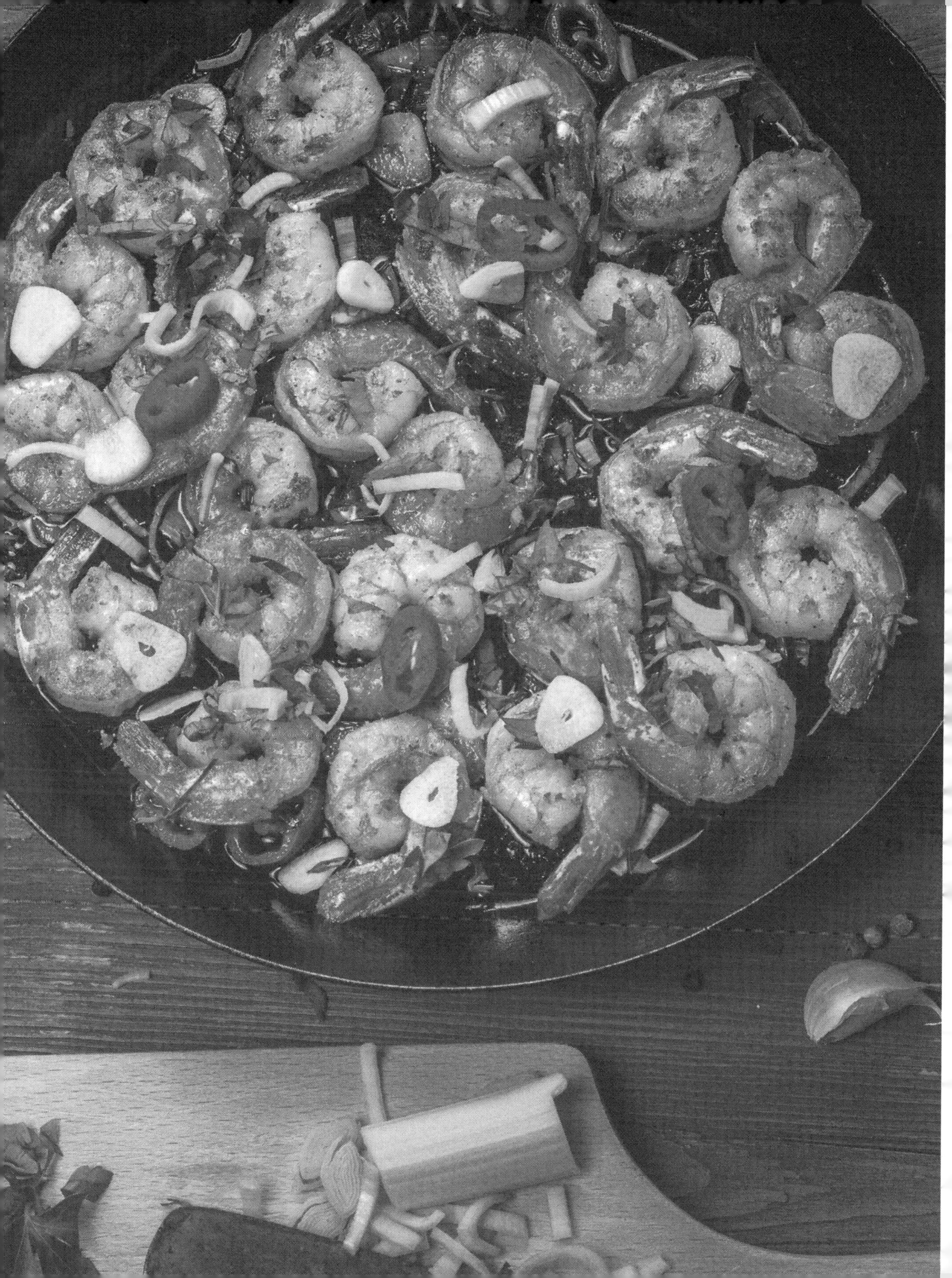

EGGS BENEDICT WITH HOLLANDAISE SAUCE WITH AVOCADO

servings: 2 | calories: 900

Ingredients

- 2 english muffin, halved
- 4 eggs, poached
- 4 slices ham, fried
- 1 ripe avocado
- 1 cup hollandaise sauce

Directions

1. Fry ham slices in vegetable oil until crispy. Drain excess grease on paper towels.
2. Toast muffins in ham fat until golden brown and crisp on both sides. Plate muffins (two for each person) and top with a slice of ham.
3. Bring an inch of water to simmer in a large, thick bottomed pan. Add a pinch of salt and 2 teaspoons white vinegar. Crack a single egg into a shallow cup and gently lower into water. Repeat until all three eggs have entered the water.
4. Turn off the heat and cover eggs for five minutes. After five minutes, remove the eggs with a slotted spoon and drain briefly on paper towels, then place each egg on top of a muffin.
5. Cut open an avocado and slice into four equal pieces with a butter knife. Scoop out with a spoon and top each egg with a slice of avocado.
6. Pour 1/4 cup of warm hollandaise sauce over each egg, serve.

There's nothing better than the traditional eggs Benedict for breakfast, especially when combined with the delicious and nutritious avocado. Pairing the richness of the hollaindaise, toasty English muffins, runny eggs, and creamy avocado is great tasting and great for you, packed with protein, fiber, and potassium to help you start your day right.

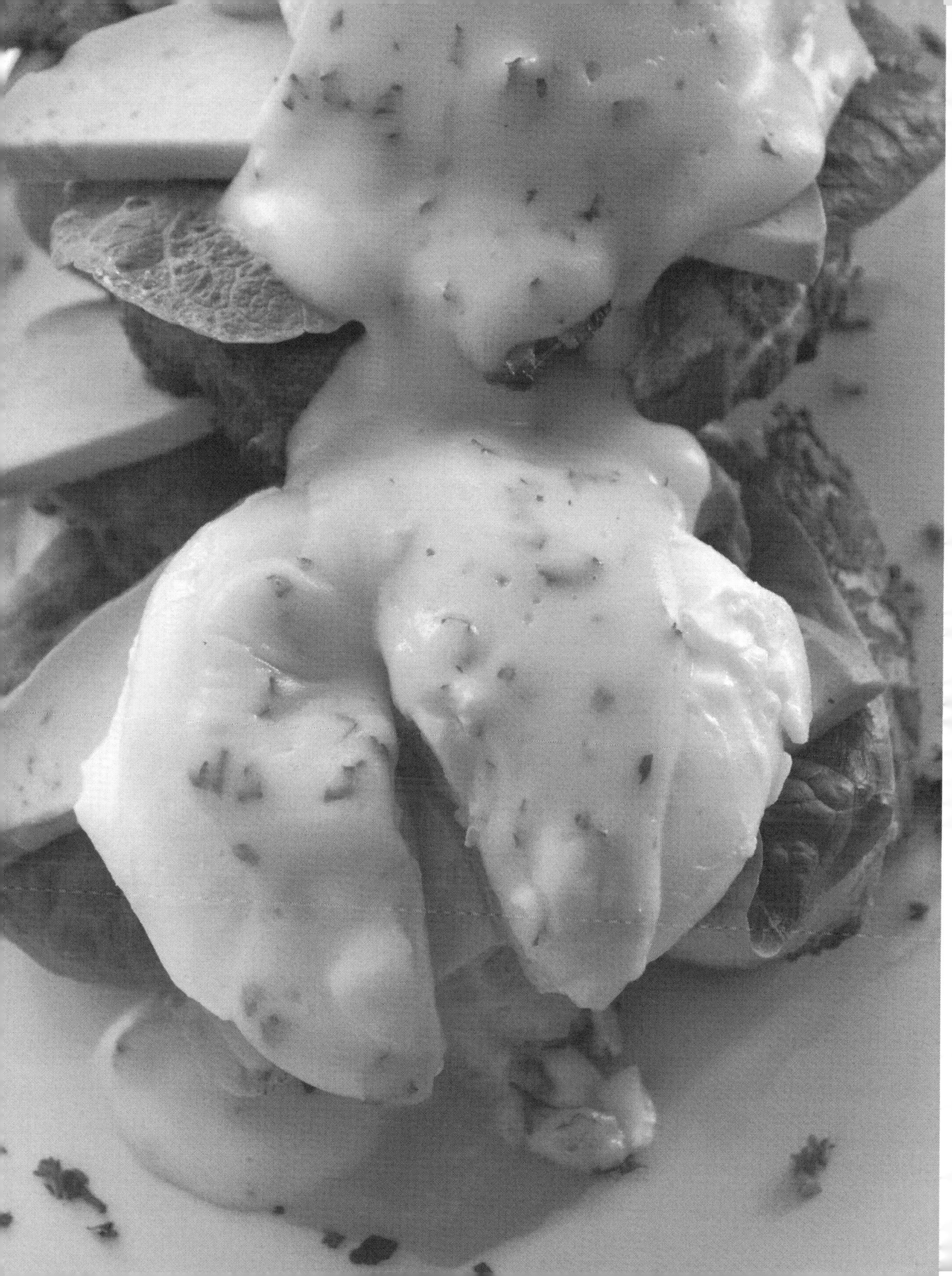

PUMPKIN SOUP IN A BOWL WITH COCONUT CREAM

servings: 4 | calories: 350

Ingredients

- 1 tbsp coconut oil
- 1 cup carrots, chopped
- 1 cup celery, chopped
- 1/2 cup onion, diced
- 1 garlic clove, minced
- 4 cups fresh pumpkin, pureed
- 2 cups vegetable broth
- 2 tsps himalayan pink salt
- 1 tsp freshly ground pepper
- 2 cups coconut cream

Directions

1. Sauté vegetables in coconut oil until they are translucent. Add garlic and sauté one minute longer. Add pumpkin puree, vegetable broth, salt, pepper, and coconut cream. Stir until they are combined. Bring the soup to a boil.
2. Reduce heat to medium-low and simmer the soup for 15 minutes before serving it.

Autumn is quickly approaching, and pumpkin lovers are rejoicing! Be sure to add this healthy Coconut Cream and Fresh Pumpkin Soup to your autumn recipes repertoire! The fresh pumpkin is loaded with vitamins A, C, and K, and the coconut cream provides necessary, healthy fat.

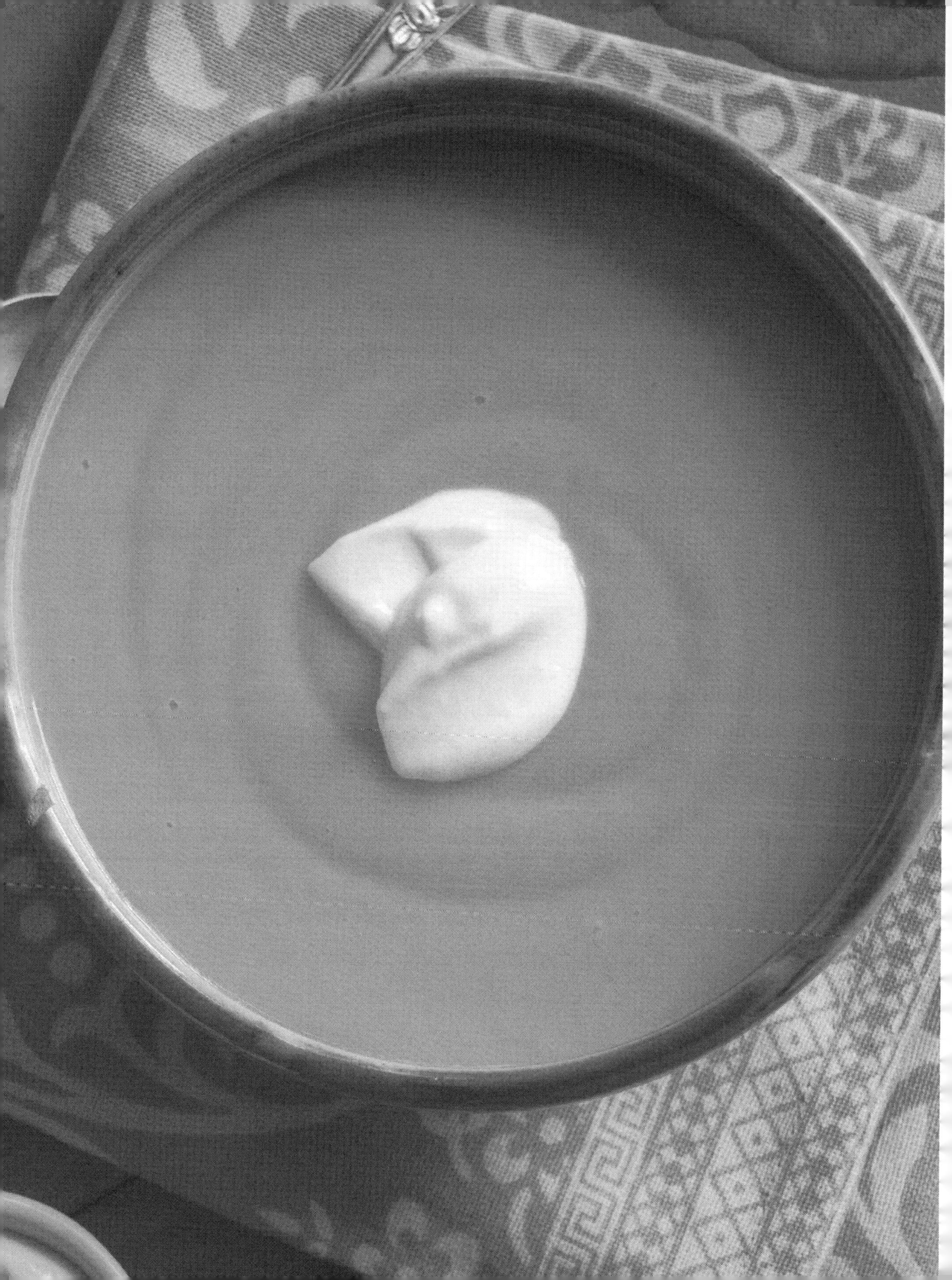

CREAMY SQUASH SOUP WITH ROSEMARY AND PAPRIKA

cooking time: 1 hr | servings: 4 - 6 | calories: 90

Ingredients

- 1 butternut squash-halved and seeded
- 1 tablespoon paprika
- 1 tablespoon olive oil
- 4 cups chicken broth

Directions

1. Preheat oven to 350
2. Baste the squash with olive oil and paprika and bake face down for 45 minutes
3. Carve squash flesh and add to a blender with the chicken broth
4. Heat purée over medium heat until thickened then serve with garnishes
5. Note: You can also include any garnishing you'd like. Popular garnishes include chives, sour cream, yogurt, or cilantro.

This healthy winter dish offers a burst of flavor and a host of health benefits. Squash is known to have high levels of beta carotene which is beneficial for eye strength and health. The broth-based nature of this dish also makes it low calorie, yet filling.

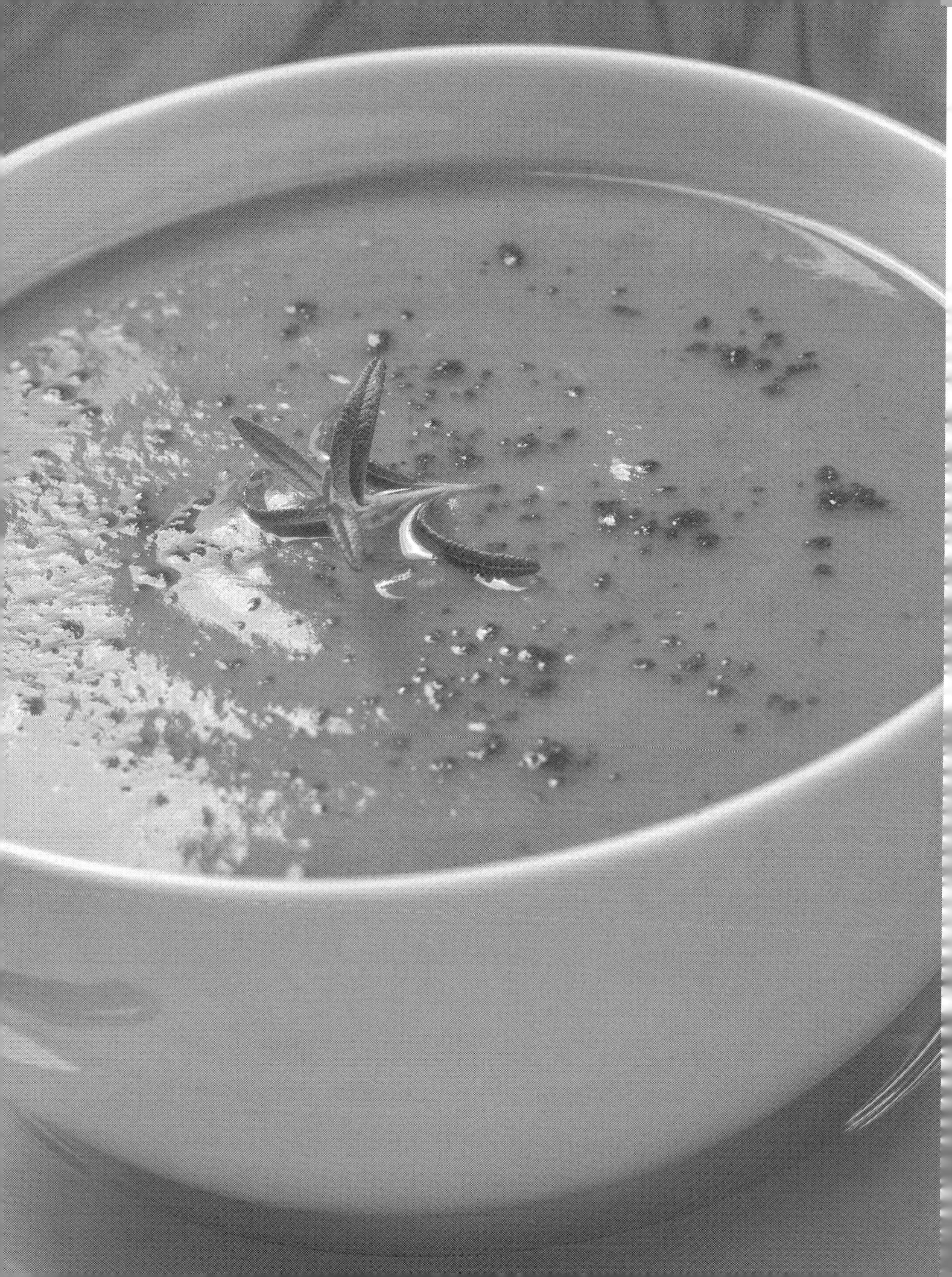

TOM YUM SOUP
A THAI TRADITIONAL SPICY PRAWN SOUP

servings: 4 | calories: 285

Ingredients

- 12 jumbo prawns (size 16/20)
- 12 oyster or shiitake mushrooms - (cut into halves)
- soba noodles, ramen noodles, or egg noodles
- 2 1/2 cups water
- 1 stalk lemongrass (whites only, pounded)
- 10 - 12 kaffir lime leaves - (pounded)
- 8 - 10, 1/4-inch galangal root - slices
- 1 small tomato (cut into quarters)
- 3 tbsps nam prik pao (thai chili paste)
- 1 tbsp fish sauce (to taste)
- 3 tbsps lime juice (fresh)
- 1/2 tsp chili powder (to taste)
- 1/2 cup cilantro (for garnish)

Directions

1. Bring a pot of water to boil. Prepare noodles, drain, and rinse with cold water. Set aside.
2. Now in the pot, bring 2 and ½ cups of water to boil. Add the aromatics to the broth--lemongrass, lime leaves, tomato, and galangal. Boil for 5-7 minutes.
3. Add shrimp, mushrooms, and nam prik phao. Continue to boil until shrimp is pink and cooked through.
4. Add the fish sauce and chili powder.
5. Remove from heat and add lime juice.
6. Build the soup in individual bowls--add noodles and ladle soup on top. Serve with fresh lime wedges and cilantro

One of the most famous and popular dishes in Thailand is Tom Yum Soup. Fresh galangal root is a natural anti-inflammatory and has been used to aid digestion, stomach pain, and rheumatoid arthritis. Tom Yum Soup is a dish that's not only delicious but also makes for a healthy and nutritious weeknight meal.

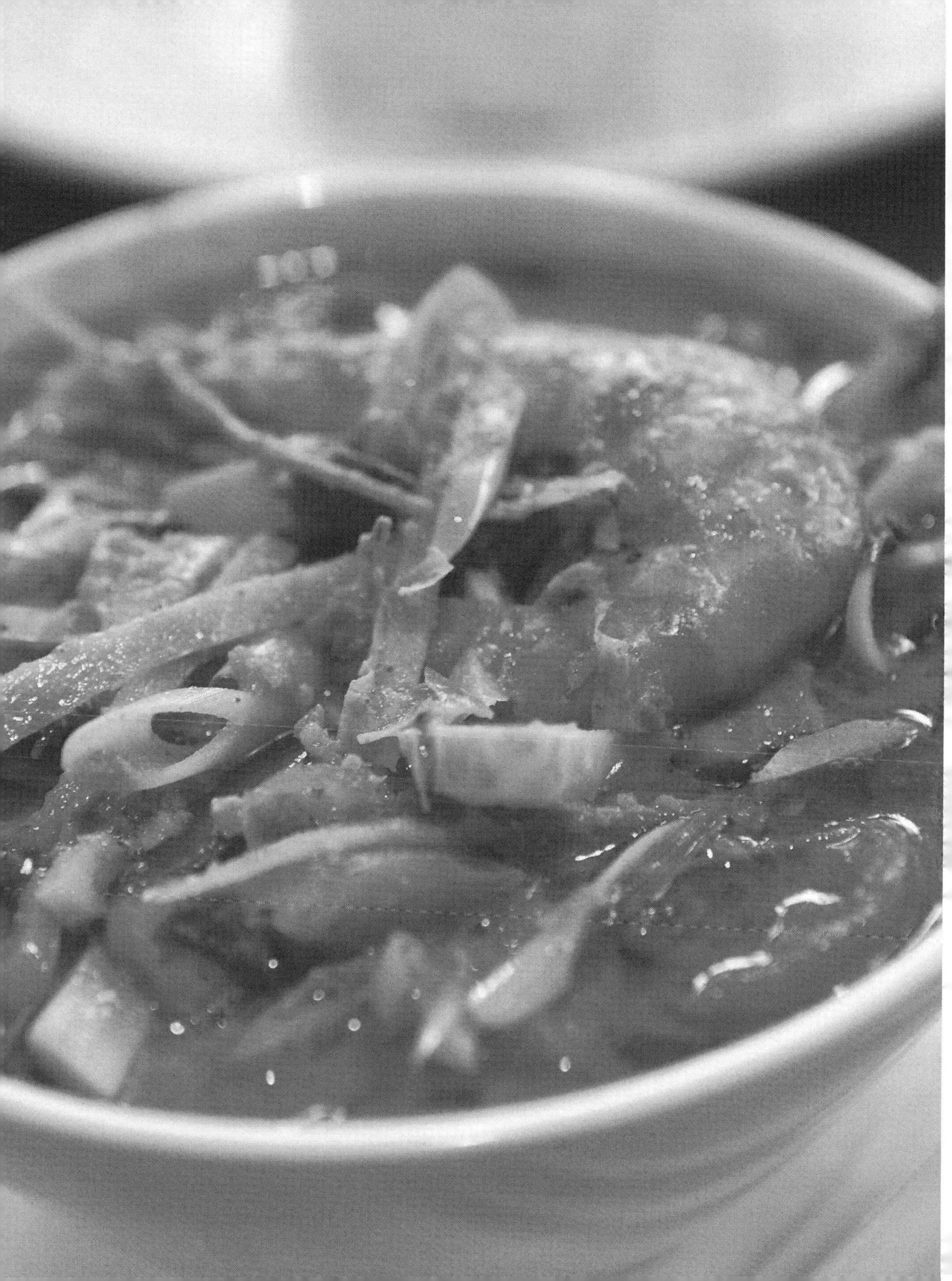

PALEO BREAD

servings: 12 | calories: 300

Ingredients

- 1 cup of almond flour
- 3/4 cup of arrowroot flour
- 1/3 cup of coconut oil, unmelted
- 1/2 cup of golden milled flax meal
- 1/4 cup of water
- 4 medium sized eggs
- 2 tbsp of maple syrup
- 1/2 tsp of sea salt
- 1 tsp of apple cider vinegar
- 2 tsps of baking soda

Directions

1. Preheat oven to 350 degrees. Place oven safe parchment paper on bread pan. Add all ingredients to food processor or blender. Once mixed, pour your batter into the bread pan and bake for 35 minutes. Top should be golden.

This recipe for paleo bread makes 12 slices, or 12 servings. Each serving is approximately 300 calories. This would make a great light breakfast option, smothered in honey butter or your favorite jam. Paleo bread is a healthy alternative to regular bread due to it being homemade and free from unnecessary added ingredients.

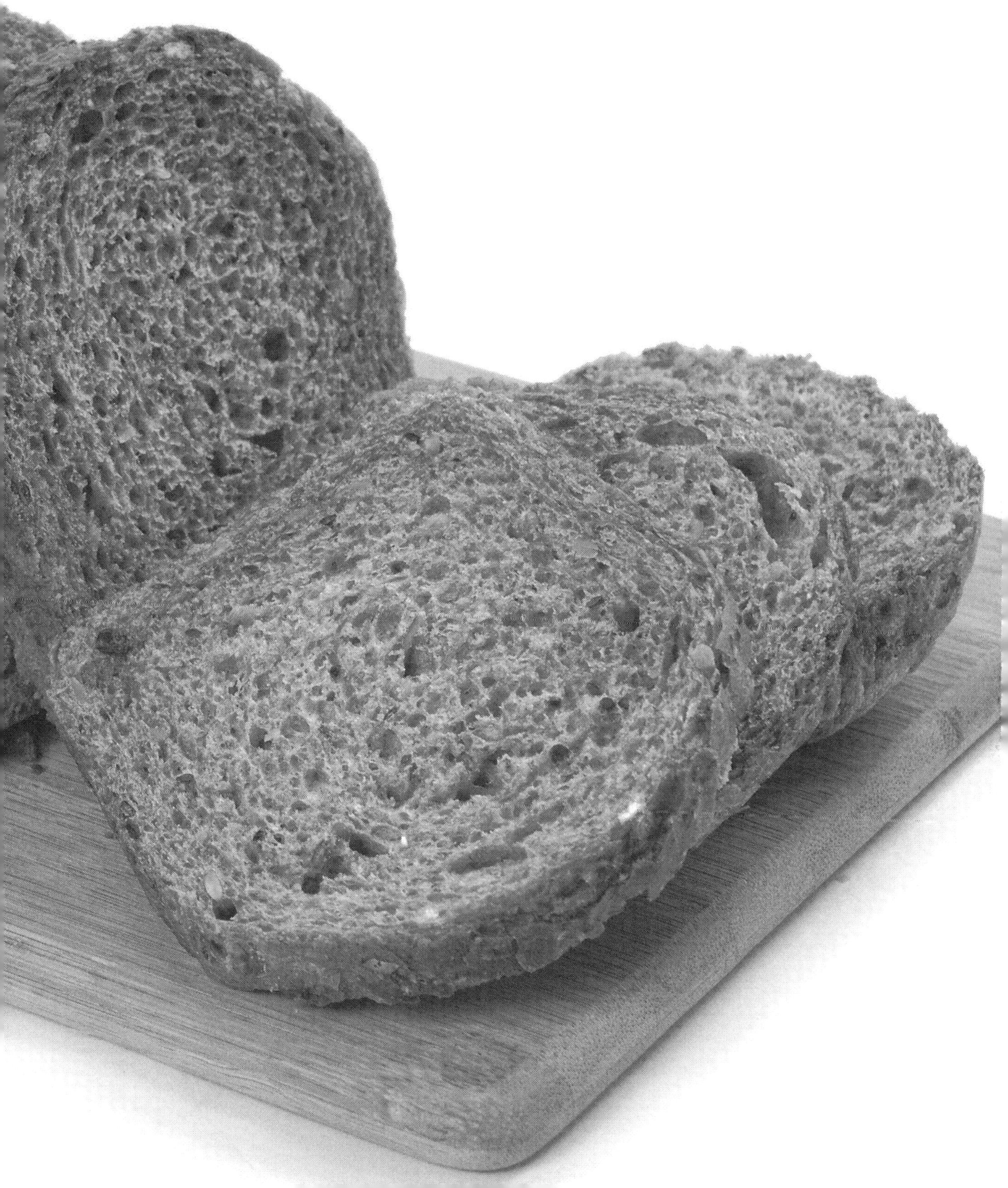

HOMEMADE CREAMY BROCCOLI SOUP

servings: 4 | calories: 120

Ingredients

- 4 cups, bite-sized (chopped) broccoli florets
- 1/2 can cream of chicken
- 1 cup coconut milk (unsweetened)
- 1/2 cup half and half
- 1/8 cup coconut flour
- spray olive oil
- sea salt and pepper to taste.

Directions

Option one:

1. In a small pan, spray olive oil to cook the broccoli florets in low heat. Use one tablespoon of the cream of chicken to wet the florets so they can start cooking with flavor.
2. In low heat, add coconut milk, the rest of the cream of chicken, and the half and half. As you add the coconut flour, be sure to whisk vigorously to mix all ingredients.

Option two:

3. Using a blender, mix together the broccoli, flour, and creams. Pour in a small pan, at low heat, and slowly add the milk, whisking as you go. Taste for salt and pepper and continue cooking (and whisking) at low heat for 10-15 minutes. Serve warm!

This healthier version of the original contains fresh broccoli florets, cream of chicken, half and half and coconut flour. It lowers the calories and the starch content for a much better digestion.

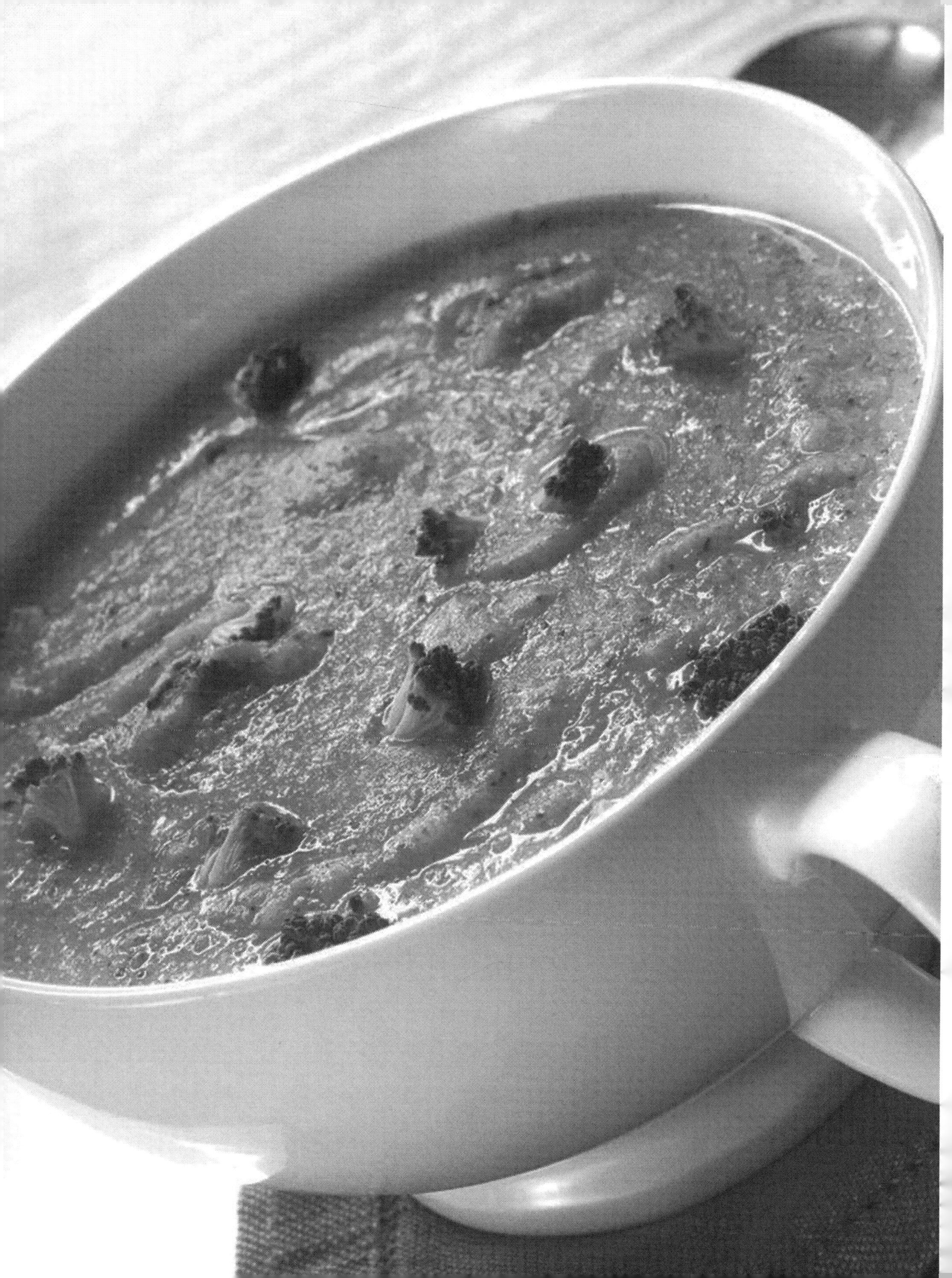

HOMEMADE PUMPKIN SOUP WITH PUMPKIN SEEDS

servings: 4 - 5 | calories: 208

Ingredients

- 1 cup canned pumpkin (not pumpkin pie filling)
- 1 1/2 cups low-sodium chicken broth
- 1/4 tsp ground ginger
- 1/8 tsp salt
- 1 tbsp butter or margarine
- 1 tbsp all-purpose flour
- 1 cup light cream (see note)
- 1/2 cup pumpkin seeds, shelled and lightly toasted

Directions

1. In a medium saucepan, stir flour, butter, ginger and salt over medium heat. Add cream, stir and cook until thickened, about 2 to 3 minutes.
2. Add chicken broth and pumpkin, stirring to mix thoroughly and heat through. Soup may be thinned with more cream if necessary.
3. Spoon soup into bowls and sprinkle with pumpkin seeds to garnish.

Note: May substitute milk for a lower-calorie soup or half-and-half for a richer soup. Calorie counts will vary.

Full of good things such as vitamins E and B6, iron, magnesium, phosphorus and fiber, pumpkin is not just for pies.

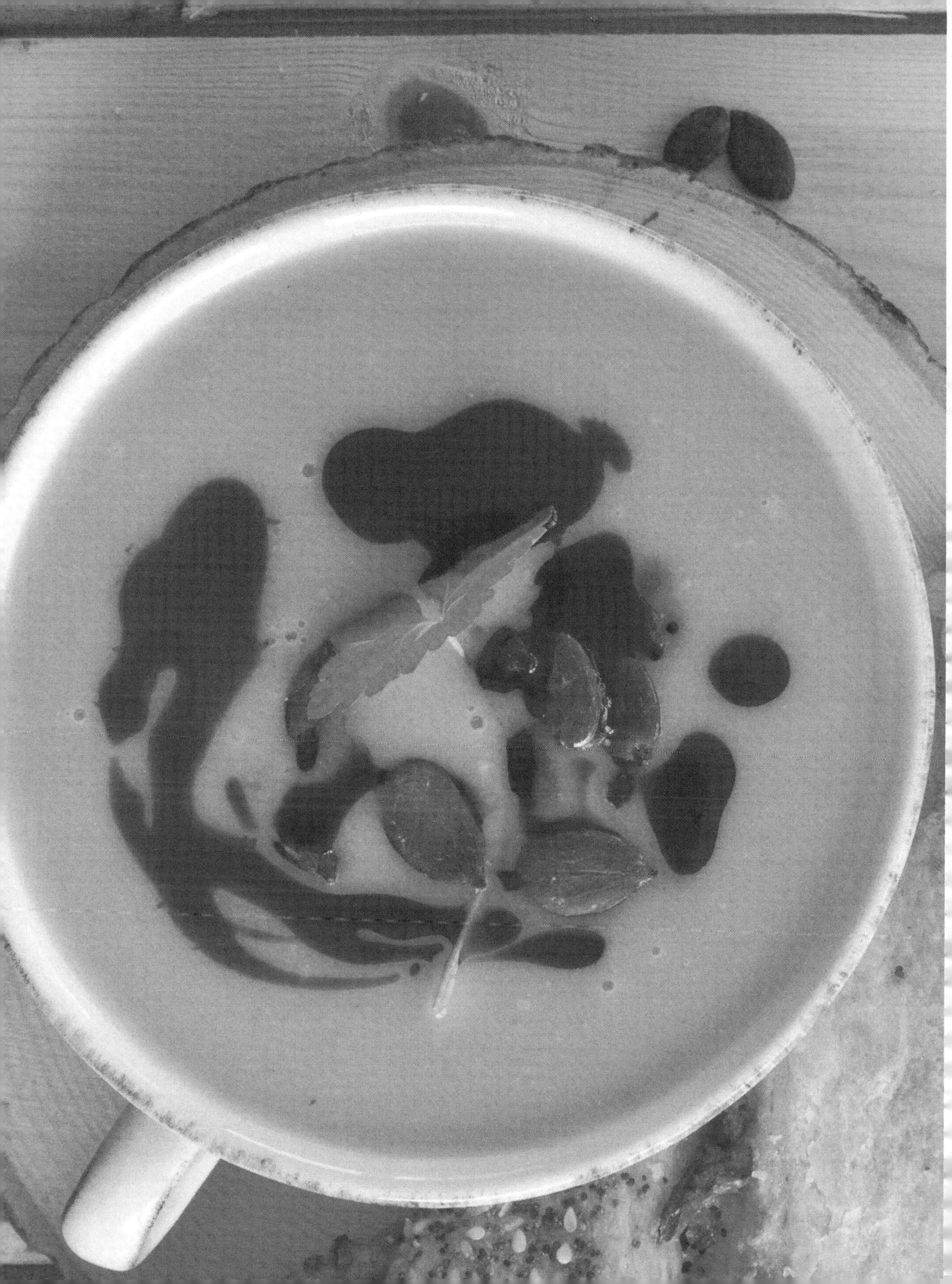

CREAMY MUSHROOM SOUP

servings: 6 | calories: 310

Ingredients

- 1 diced up onion
- 1 1/2 lbs of thinly sliced cremini mushrooms
- 1/4 cup butter
- 3 cloves garlic, minced
- 4 cups chicken broth
- 1 cup red wine
- 1/2 tsp dried thyme
- 1 cup heavy cream
- 2 tbsp cornstarch
- preferred amounts of black pepper and salt to taste

Directions

1. In a larch stockpot melt your butter. Next, add mushrooms and garlic and stir occasionally. Once browned, season pan with pepper and salt. Stir in the onion until tender. At this point, add the wine and bring to a boil.
2. Simmer at lower heat until the wine has been slightly reduced. Introduce thyme, heavy cream, and chicken broth. Whisk 1/4 water with the cornstarch in separate bowl. Stir this mix into the soup until thick.
3. Cook until prepared - add more salt and pepper to taste.

A unique creamy mushroom soup that's full of healthy ingredients, this recipe yields 6 servings and each serving is 310 calories. Mushrooms are great for helping the body in producing vitamin D and iron. Mushrooms are also a healthy way to fill yourself on a low calorie diet.

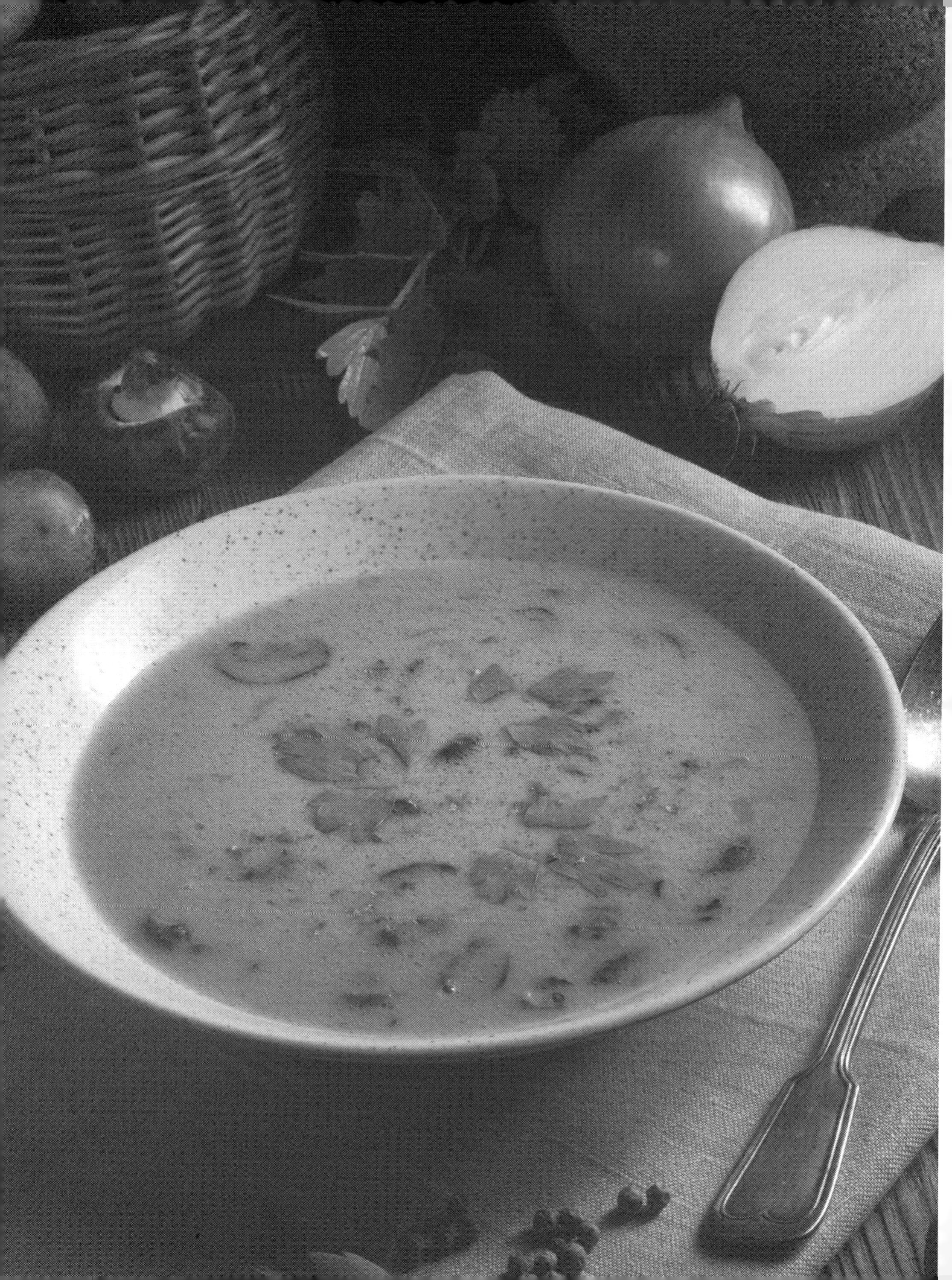

HOMEMADE BEEF SOUP WITH VEGETABLES

servings: 10 | calories: 268

Ingredients

- 1 pound of ground beef
- 1 16 once box of chicken broth

Vegetables:

- 1 frozen package of cocktail onions
- 6 diced fresh potatoes
- 5 sliced fresh carrots
- 1 15 oz. can sweet yellow kernel corn
- 2 cups fresh green beans cut in half
- 1 cup of fresh celery

Seasonings:

- 1 tablespoon of salt
- 1 teaspoon of pepper
- 2 tablespoon of worcestershire sauce

Directions

1. Sprinkle ground beef with salt, pepper and Worcestershire sauce
2. (if time permits, place in the refrigerator from 30 minutes to overnight for greater desired taste intensity)
3. Brown the beef in a large pot over medium to high heat. Remove the ground beef from the pan without draining or disturbing the residue that remains in the pot
4. Place the ground beef on a paper plate covered with paper towels to drain all of the fat from the meat. Stir to loosen residue that is at the bottom of the pot (this will intensify flavor)
5. Add ground beef back to the pot. Stir the loosened residue into the ground beef. Add all vegetables and chicken broth to the pot. Stir and mix very well. Bring your uncovered pot to a roaring boil. Add cover and simmer for 45-1 hour) (until the potatoes are tender)
6. Reduce temperature from simmer to warm. Serve bowls as requested
7. Suggestion: Cut all vegetables approximately the same size for even cooking

This delicious homemade beef soup with vegetables is a warm, hearty comfort food. A great dish for a group of 8-10 people who are eating at different times and helping themselves.

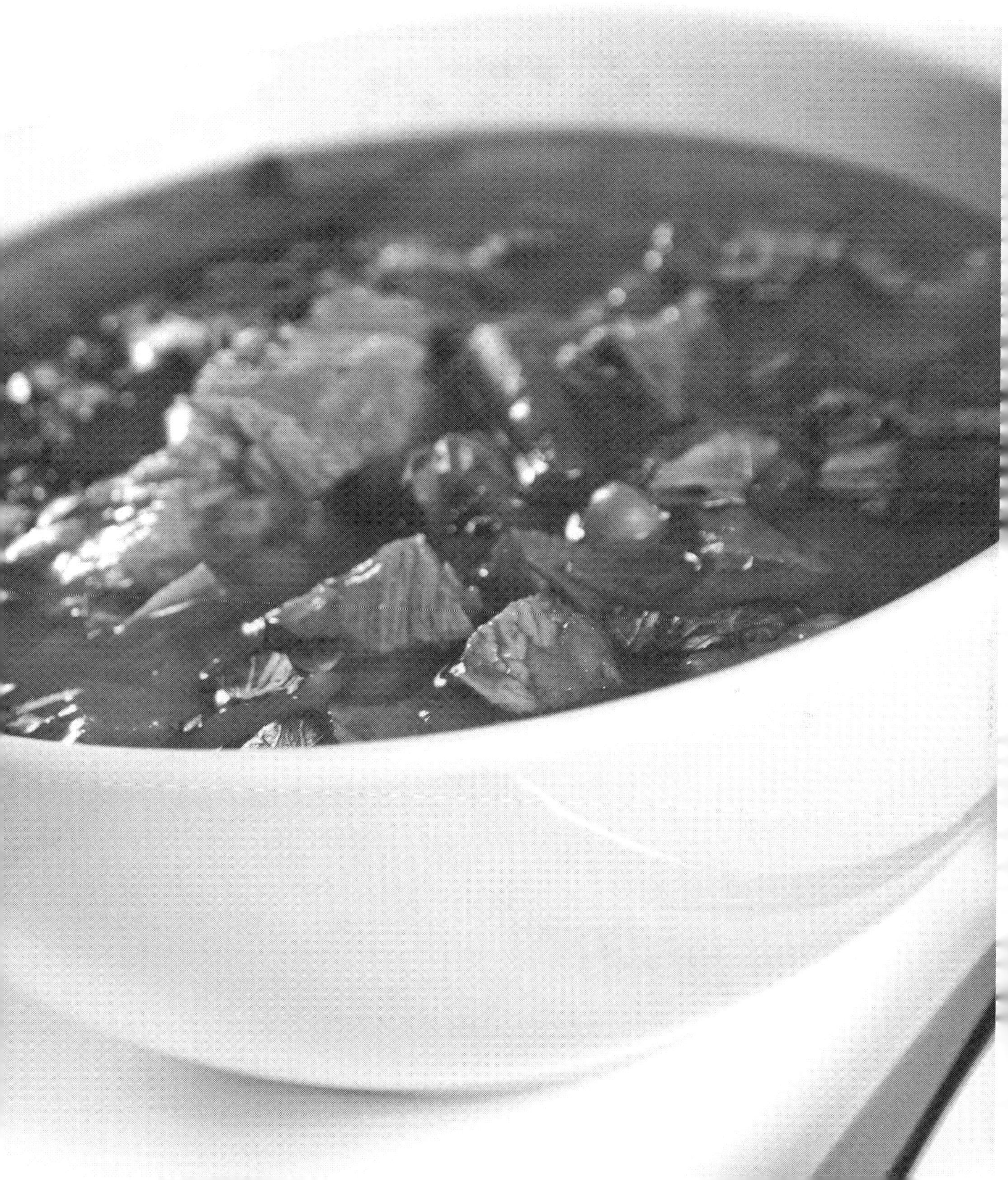

HOMEMADE ONION SOUP WITH CELERY

servings: 8 | calories: 108

Ingredients

- 1 tablespoon of butter (not margarine)
- 3 cups diced celery
- 3 cups diced sweet onion, like a Vidalia
- 2 tables of fresh thyme, cut finely
- 7 cloves of fresh garlic, minced
- 4 cups of homemade or unsalted canned chicken stock
- 2 cups water
- Salt and freshly-cracked pepper-to taste
- 1-inch slice of lemon rind
- 1 slice of stale French bread-cubed
- 1/4 cup buttermilk
- Optional toppings: A tablespoon of sour cream sprinkled with chives

Directions

1. Melt the butter in a heavy soup pot over medium heat. Watch it carefully, because butter burns easily. Add the onion, celery, garlic, and thyme. Cover the pot and gently cook for about 20 minutes, until the onions are transparent and the celery is tender. Stir occasionally during cooking time.
2. Add water, chicken stock, and lemon rind to the mixture, and simmer for another 20 minutes. Discard the lemon rind.
3. Next, add the stale bread cubes and stir the mixture well.
4. Pour about half of the mixture in a blender, and secure the lid. Be sure to take the middle cap out of the blender lid so steam can escape safely. Cover the top with a clean dish towel, and puree mixture until smooth. Pour mixture into a large bowl, and repeat step with the remaining mixture. Pour the pureed soup back into your soup pot.
5. Turn up the stove to medium heat and add the buttermilk. Stir the soup until it is hot, but not boiling. Serve in bowls or mugs with a dollop of sour cream and sprinkled chives.

What could be more comforting than a steaming bowl of fragrant onion and celery soup! Onions are chock full of antioxidants that can ward off disease. The addition of celery gives this soup a creamy zest.

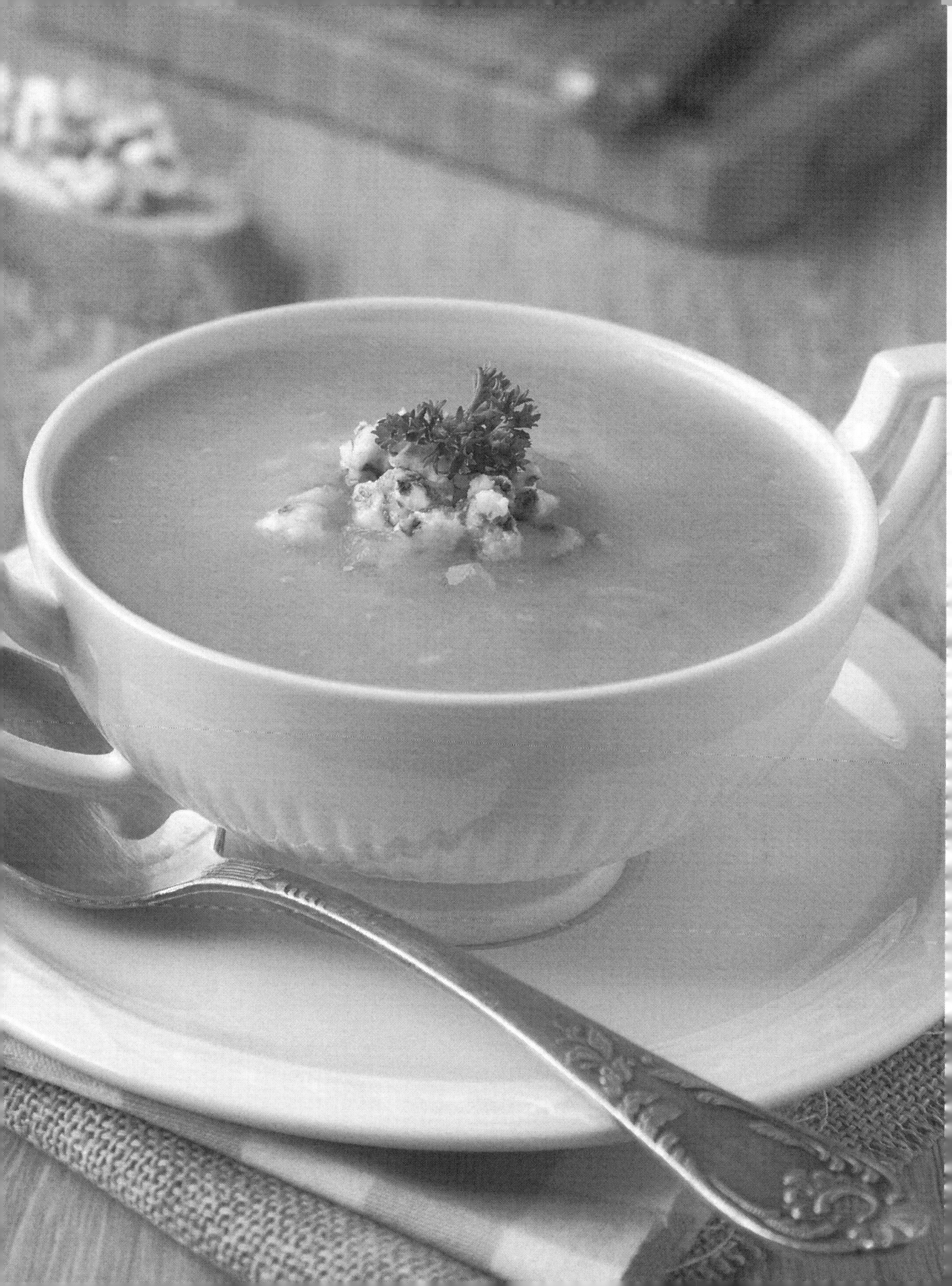

RATATOUILLE

servings: 4 | calories: 200

Ingredients

- 1/2 cup shredded basil leaves
- 3/4 tsp salt
- 1/8 tsp ground coriander
- 1/4 tsp fennel seeds
- 1/4 tsp dried thyme, crumbled
- 3/4 lb small ripe tomatoes, chopped
- 1/4 tsp dried oregano
- 1 small zucchini, cut in thin slices
- 1 red bell pepper, chopped
- 3/4 lb eggplant, cut into 1/2 in pieces
- 2 garlic cloves, minced
- 1 whole onion, sliced thinly
- 2 garlic cloves
- 5 tbsps olive oil

Directions

1. Using 2 tbsp olive oil, cook onion and garlic in large skillet. After, add in remaining 3 tbsp olive oil and add in eggplant, occasionally stirring. Then, stir in zucchini, tomatoes, and bell pepper and cook until soft. Add all other ingredients and stir frequently. Cook on medium for 5 minutes.
2. Ratatouille may be prepared the day before serving for best results. Refrigerate covered.

Ratatouille is full of dietary fiber, vitamin B6, and Potassium. It's very low in cholesterol and sodium.

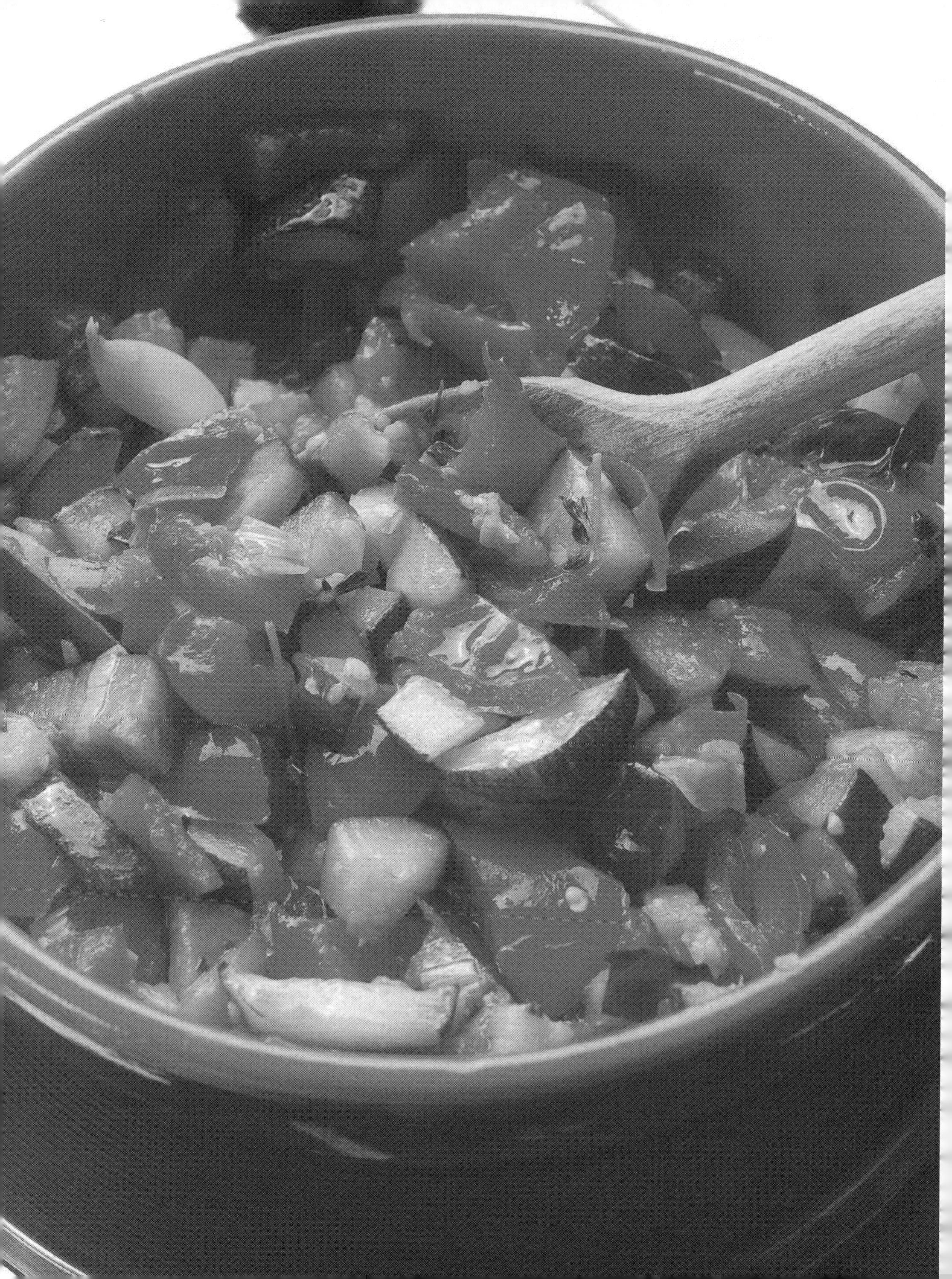

ROASTED CHICKEN LEG WITH POTATOES

servings: 4

Ingredients

- 2 lbs chicken legs
- 2 lbs potatoes cut into quarters
- 4 garlic cloves, peeled
- fresh herbs – rosemary, sage, thyme
- 4 tbsps extra virgin olive oil
- salt and pepper to taste

Directions

1. Season the chicken with salt and pepper. Sprinkle the herbs on and around the chicken. Drizzle the olive oil over the meat. Stir to coat all pieces in oil, herbs, salt, and pepper. Let the chicken marinate in the refrigerator for 30 minutes.
2. While the chicken is marinating, season the potatoes with salt and pepper. Set them aside.
3. Preheat the oven to 375F.
4. Place the chicken, potatoes, and garlic in a casserole dish and bake for 20 minutes.
5. Remove the dish from the oven and turn the chicken and potatoes.
6. Return to dish to the oven to bake for another 20-30 minutes.
7. When the deepest part of the flesh is pierced with a skewer and the juices run clear, the chicken is done.

This healthy meal can be in the oven in 30 minutes and on the plates in another 40 minutes. It's sure to be a winner with your family.

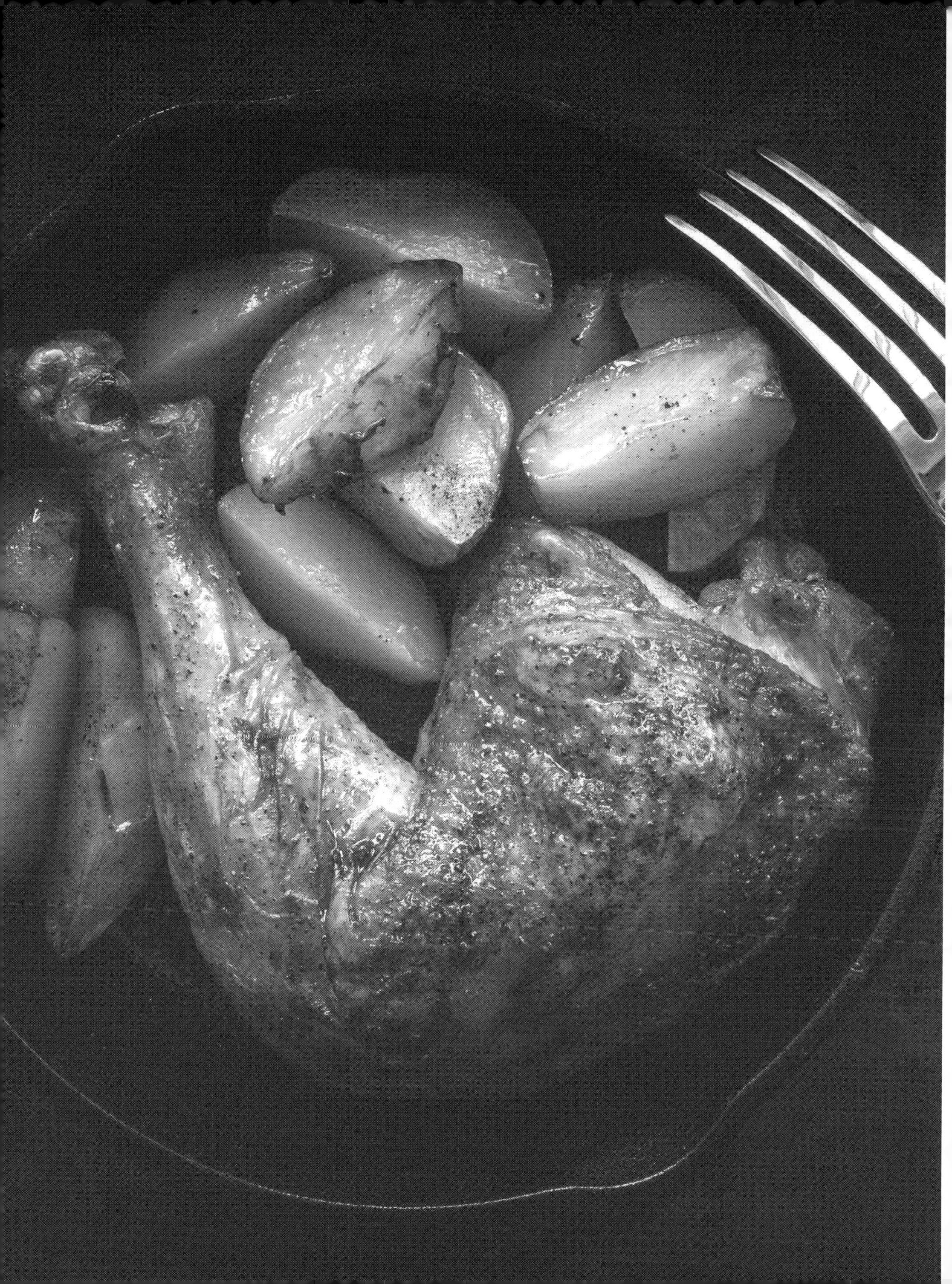

ROASTED CHICKEN

servings: 8 | calories: 180

Ingredients

- 1 whole chicken

Seasonings:

- 1 tsp of salt
- 1 tsp of pepper
- 1 tbsp garlic salt
- 1 tbsp paprika
- 1 tbsp worcestershire sauce
- 1/2 tsp of olive oil
- cooking spray

Directions

1. Preheat oven at 375 degrees F. Spray empty pan with cooking spray
2. Pat chicken dry with paper towels (this step ensures a crispy skin and moist meat). Place chicken breast up in pan. Rub olive oil into the chicken
3. Sprinkle the salt, garlic salt, pepper, paprika, and Worcestershire sauce over and inside chicken cavity
4. Place chicken into the oven
5. Baste chicken with juices found inside the pan every 20 minutes
6. Cook chicken for 1 1/2 hours
7. Let chicken stand for 10 minutes before carving and serving

This delicious roasted chicken recipe is a simple, tasty comfort food that's perfect as a weekly dish. It is high in protein yet low-fat and low-calorie enough to be a perfect addition to a weight maintenance menu.

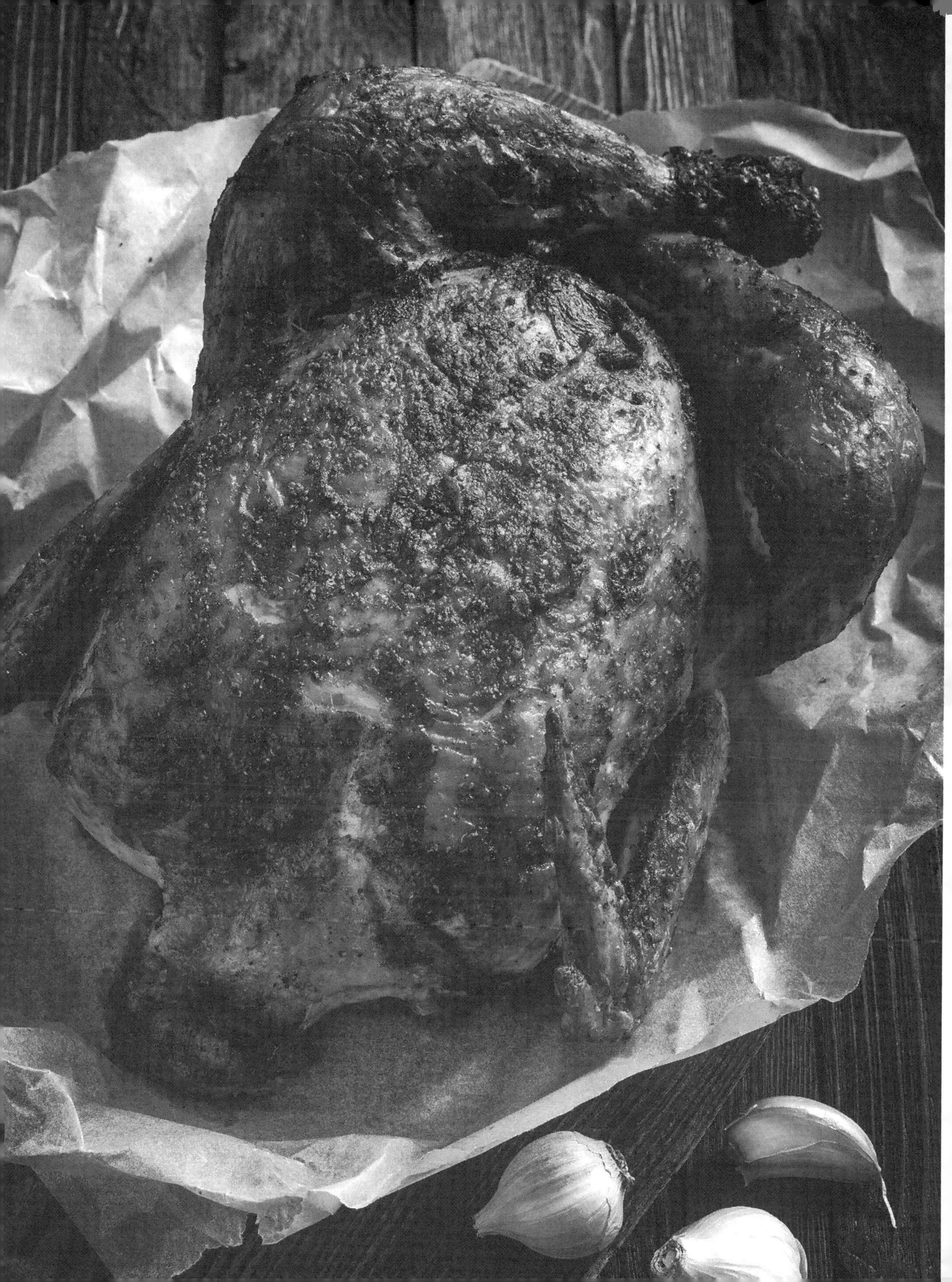

BARBECUED RIBS SEASONED WITH A SPICY BASTING SAUCE

servings: 4 | calories: 500

Ingredients

- 2 - 2 lbs racks of baby back ribs
- 1 tbsp jerk seasoning
- 1 cup dark or spiced rum

Directions

1. Take two 2-pound racks of baby back ribs, rinse, and leave to dry.
2. Rub 1 tablespoon of jerk seasoning blend into the ribs evenly.
3. Pour 1 cup of dark or spiced rum into a shallow dish , and add the ribs, turning regularly to coat the entire surface. Allow the ribs to chill for one hour, still turning occasionally.
4. Use one side of the grill and heat to between 325-350 degrees fahrenheit, placing a drip pan beneath the side that is not used. Put ribs on this side.
5. Grill for 2.5-3 hours or until ribs are tender and the bones are showing.
6. Brush with 1/2 cup of rum BBQ sauce, grilling for 15 minutes.

Baby back pork ribs are perfect for summer, and even better when you have a spicy jerk sauce on top! While these ribs can be high on the calorie side, baby back ribs are packed with protein, supplying nearly forty percent of your daily nutritional value with just a single 3 ounce serving.

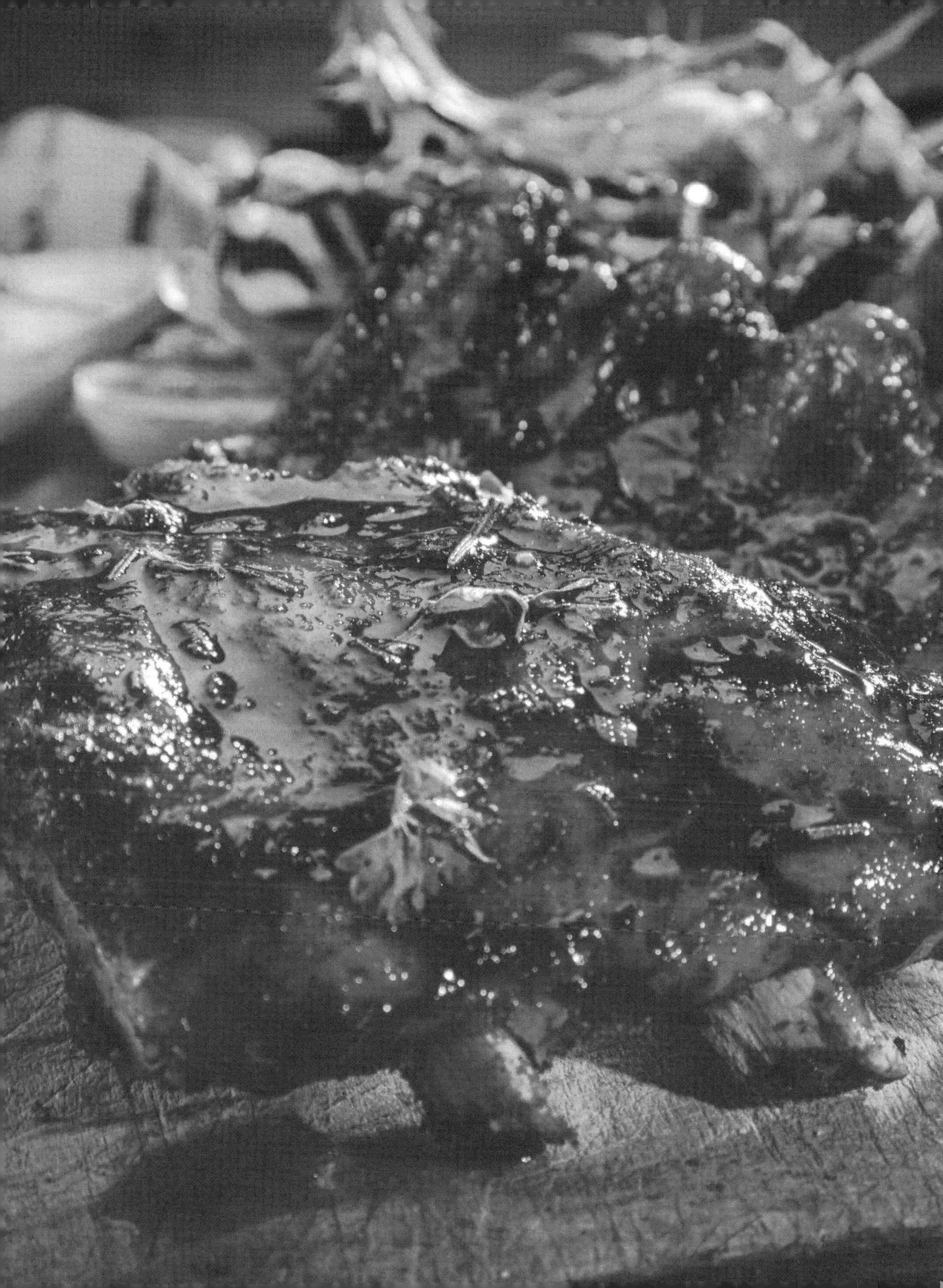

GRILLED PORK CHOPS

cooking time: 0h 0m | servings: 0 | calories: 0

Ingredients

- 6 lean pork chop loins
- 1/2 cup water
- 1/3 cup soy sauce
- 1/4 cup vegetable oil
- 3 tbsps lemon pepper
- 2 tsps garlic, minced

Directions

1. Mix all of the above spices and liquids in a deep mixing bowl. Once everything is well blended, add the pork chops and cover the bowl with plastic wrap. Let the pork chops marinate for at least 2 hours in the refrigerator. You can even let them marinate overnight for a nice deep saturation.
2. Light the grill at a medium heat and spread a light coat of vegetable oil on the grates.
3. Remove the pork chops from the mixing bowl and allow the marinate to drip off.
4. Grill the pork chops for 5 to 6 minutes per side until there is no pink in the center. Using a grilling thermometer, the center should read 145 degrees F.
5. Now you are ready to plate, serve and enjoy!

Pool parties. Days at the beach. Playing with the family at the park. We all have our own favorite things we love about summer. Another big one you can add to the list is making dinner out on the grill. Dinner just simply tastes better on the grill. You just can't beat the taste that the combination of charcoal and smoke provide.

One of the most popular choices to grill are pork chops. They are healthy alternatives to burgers and steaks. Lean pork chops contain fewer calories and grilling them allows the fat to drip away, unlike when you fry them.

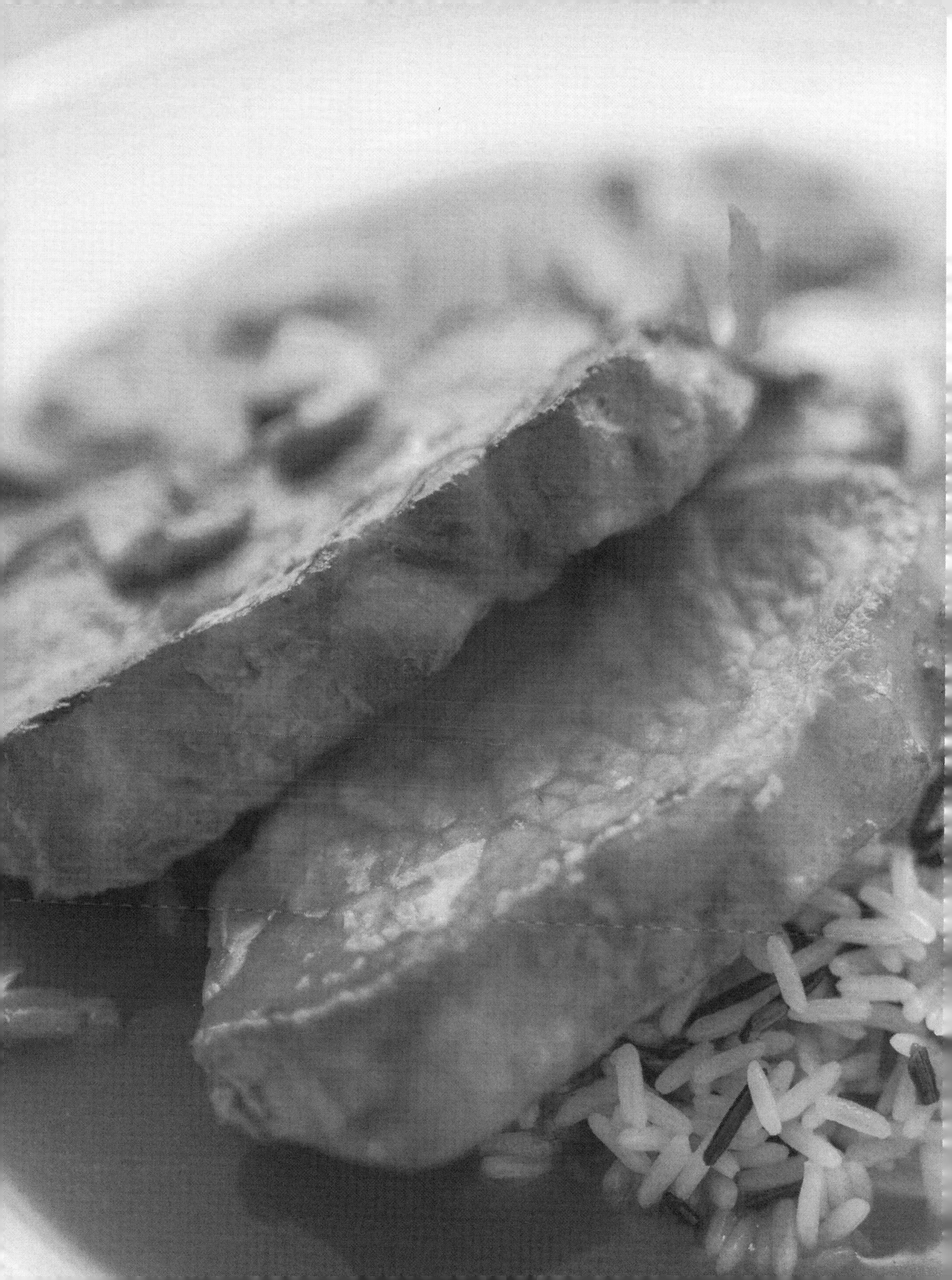

INDEX

Manufactured by Amazon.ca
Bolton, ON

10400137R00061